A Thumbnail Sketch of Theatre Nursing

A Thumbnail Sketch of Theatre Nursing

JENNIFER ANN MORRIS, SRN, SCM

Illustrations by
JANET NUNN

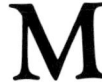

Text © Jennifer Ann Morris 1983
Illustrations © Janet Nunn 1983

All rights reserved. No part of this publication may be reproduced or transmitted, in any form or by any means, without permission.

First published 1983 by
THE MACMILLAN PRESS LTD
London and Basingstoke
Companies and representatives throughout the world

Typeset in Rockwell by Repro-type, London N13, England.

Printed in Great Britain at The Pitman Press, Bath

ISBN 0 333 35769 8 (hard cover)
     0 333 35770 1 (paper cover)

CONTENTS

Introduction viii

Acknowledgements ix

1. On First Entering Theatre 2

     Changing clothes 3
     Tour of theatre suite 5
     Policies 6

2. Reception Area 7

3. Anaesthetic Room 8

     Nurse duties: Checking 9
     Equipment 10
     Patient in anaesthetic room 16
     Patient anaesthesia 18
     Drugs used in anaesthesia 20
     Regional anaesthesia 23
     Local anaesthesia 24
     Cardiac arrest 25

4. Preparation of Theatre 26

     Circulating nurse duties 26
     Scrub nurse duties 28

CONTENTS

5. The Operation	39
Scrub nurse duties	40
Circulating nurse duties	46
Cardiac arrest	50
6. Recovery Room	52
Preparation	52
Patient in recovery room	53
Respiratory or cardiac arrest	56
7. Theatre Sterile Supply Unit	57
Instruments	59
Sutures	62/63
8. Conclusion	65
Glossary	66
Appendix: Outline of the Recommended Syllabus	67
Useful Addresses	69
Index	72

INTRODUCTION

This book is intended primarily for student nurses entering the operating theatre for the first time. In unfamiliar surroundings, with people unrecognisably hidden behind caps and masks, instant indignation if the wrong thing is touched and none of the familiar ward routines, the new staff member is every bit as anxious as the patient!

This is not intended as a definitive textbook but rather as a good humoured guide for the student nurse during the initial phase of learning theatre routine.

For the text to flow smoothly, 'student nurse' also refers to trainee operating department assistant (ODA) and auxiliaries. Also for reasons of flow, not prejudice, the nurse is usually refered to as 'she', and the doctor as 'he'. The duties of trained nurses applies equally to trained ODAs.

The book is designed to fit into the theatre uniform and can be used as a reference easily available when the nurse feels too nervous to ask questions in a busy theatre suite. For more details and for specialist procedures the nurse should avail herself of further textbooks on the theatre bookshelf.

This book is written with a number of countries in mind, including Canada, the USA and the 'developing' ones. The descriptions of scrubbing up, gowning and gloving are detailed as the student nurse may need to refer to them when practising at home. Lists of instruments have been deliberately excluded as no two surgeons use the same, finance dictates what is purchased and names vary between countries.

We are as one in the common cause of improving patient care.

Kidlington, 1983   J.A.M.

ACKNOWLEDGEMENTS

I should like to thank Miss Josephine Daly and Miss Ann Adams of The Royal Free Hospital London for their help and inspiration, and Janet Nunn whose illustrations clarify and add humour to the text.

I am grateful to my mother, Mrs Ida Morris, for painstaking typing and to the National Association of Theatre Nurses for the aims and objectives of theatre experience and the recommended syllabus.

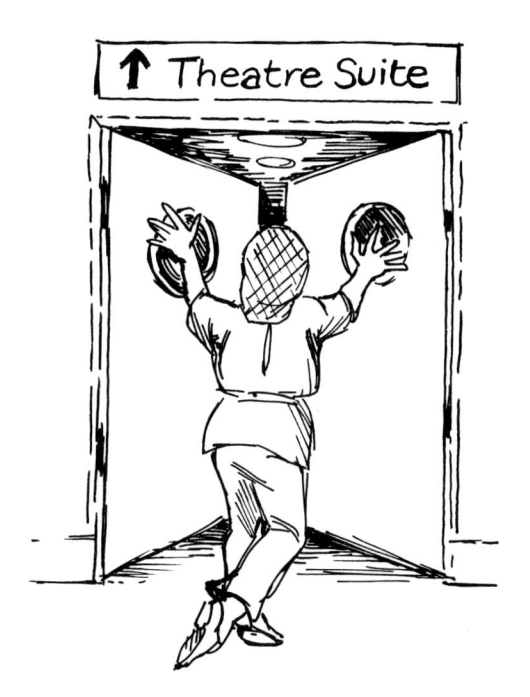

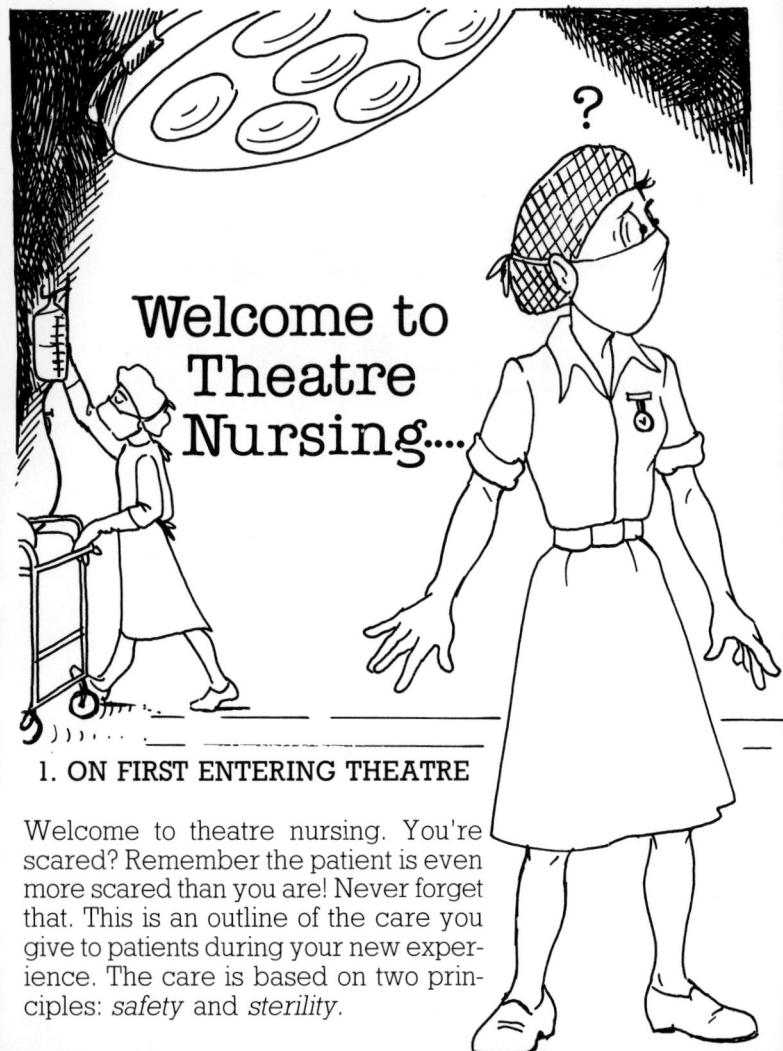

1. ON FIRST ENTERING THEATRE

Welcome to theatre nursing. You're scared? Remember the patient is even more scared than you are! Never forget that. This is an outline of the care you give to patients during your new experience. The care is based on two principles: *safety* and *sterility*.

CHANGING CLOTHES

The aim is to cut down on any bacteria brought from the outside into the clean theatre suite and so reduce the possibility of the patient getting a wound infection. Cotton uniforms are provided as cotton generates less static electricity, sparks of which could cause a fire in the presence of some anaesthetic gases. Theatre shoes have antistatic soles.

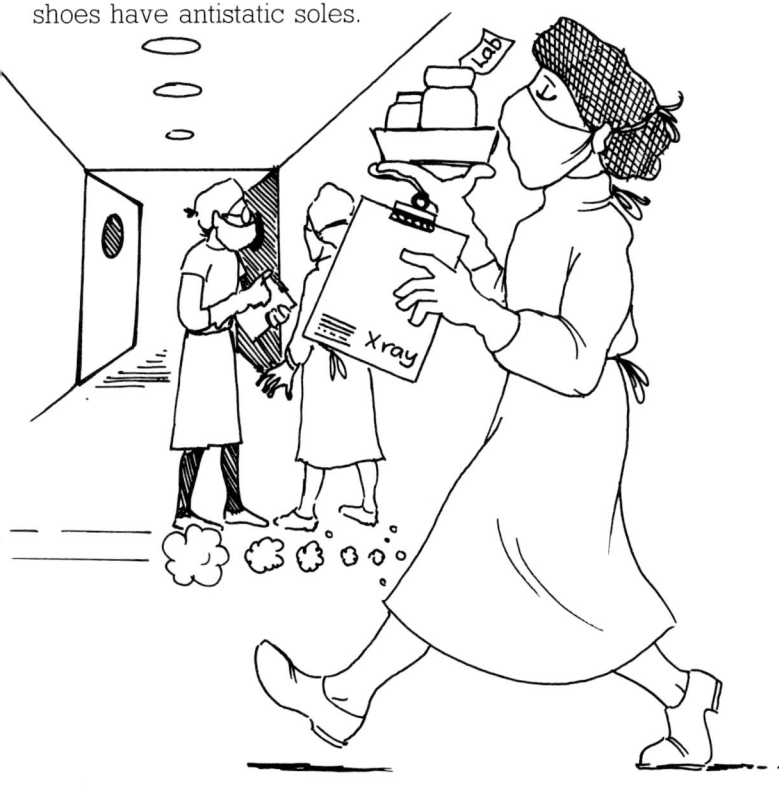

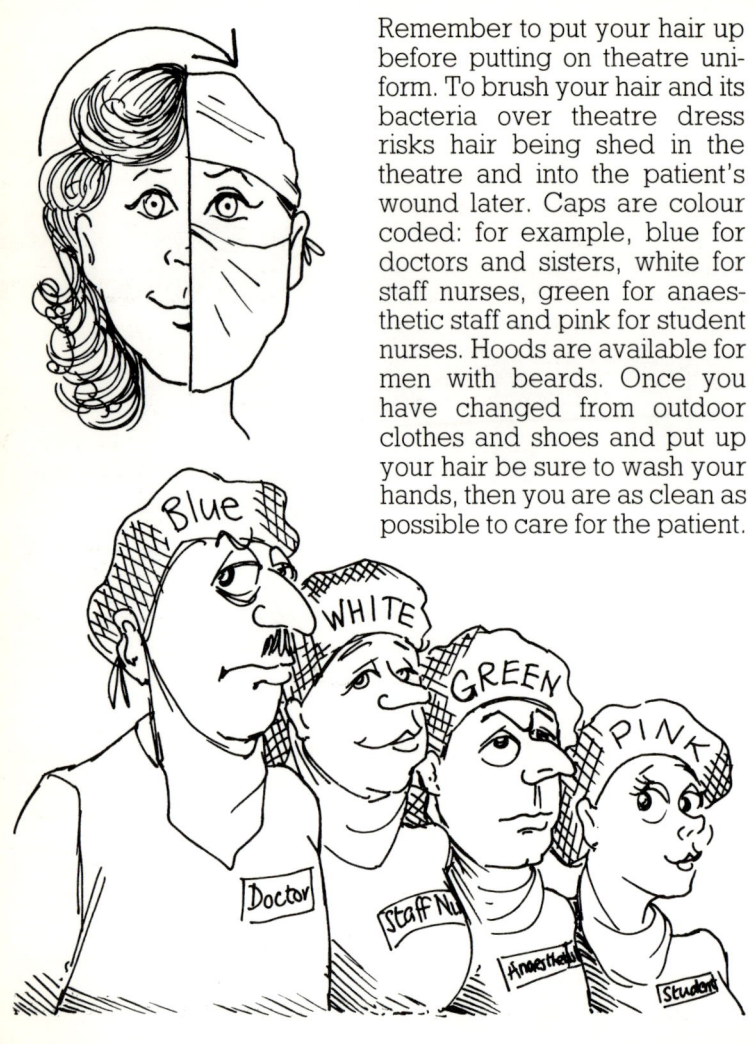

Remember to put your hair up before putting on theatre uniform. To brush your hair and its bacteria over theatre dress risks hair being shed in the theatre and into the patient's wound later. Caps are colour coded: for example, blue for doctors and sisters, white for staff nurses, green for anaesthetic staff and pink for student nurses. Hoods are available for men with beards. Once you have changed from outdoor clothes and shoes and put up your hair be sure to wash your hands, then you are as clean as possible to care for the patient.

TOUR OF THEATRE SUITE

Someone will show you round the general layout of theatres. It may seem like a confusing maze but it will get easier! Every theatre suite has a reception area, anaesthetic room, theatre itself and recovery room. There is a storage room for general supplies, an area for sterile supplies, a disposal area for used equipment, a theatre sterile supply unit (TSSU) for cleaning and sterilising; and sister's office, coffee room and changing room.

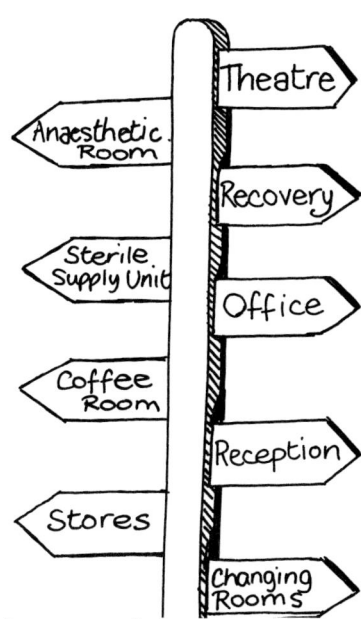

It is very important always to remember that *'IF YOU DON'T KNOW, DON'T GO.'*

If ever you are asked for anything, equipment, supplies or to take a message, and you don't understand, *stand there and say so.* The trained members of staff know exactly where to find things and can give you detailed instructions. This is quicker and means the patient isn't subjected to a longer anaesthetic and open wound while waiting for you to wander off vaguely looking for something somewhere.

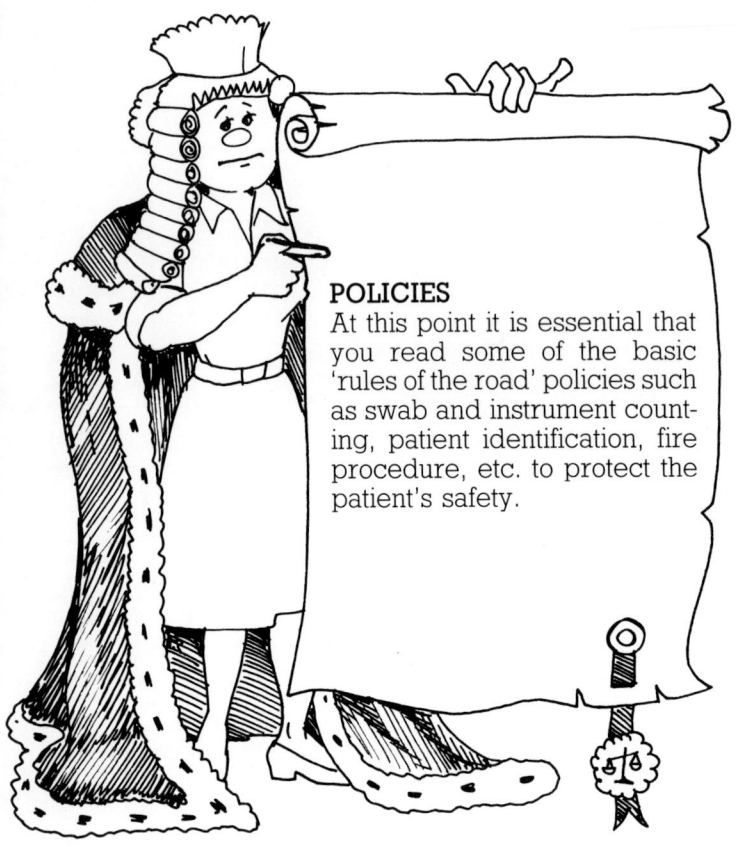

POLICIES
At this point it is essential that you read some of the basic 'rules of the road' policies such as swab and instrument counting, patient identification, fire procedure, etc. to protect the patient's safety.

The sections that follow give a more detailed description of the areas of theatre and what your duties are as part of the team caring for the patient.

2. RECEPTION AREA

Patients arrive in this area and are checked in. This is extremely important to ensure that the correct patient goes to the correct theatre for the correct procedure, accompanied by appropriate notes and X-rays. As the reception area is the patient's first encounter with theatre is it very important to give a warm welcome and to obtain all the appropriate information in a caring manner. Beds are wheeled over a 'tacky mat' to remove gross dirt. The patient is then transferred to a theatre trolley and the linen changed, again to minimise potential outside contamination of the inside clean area.

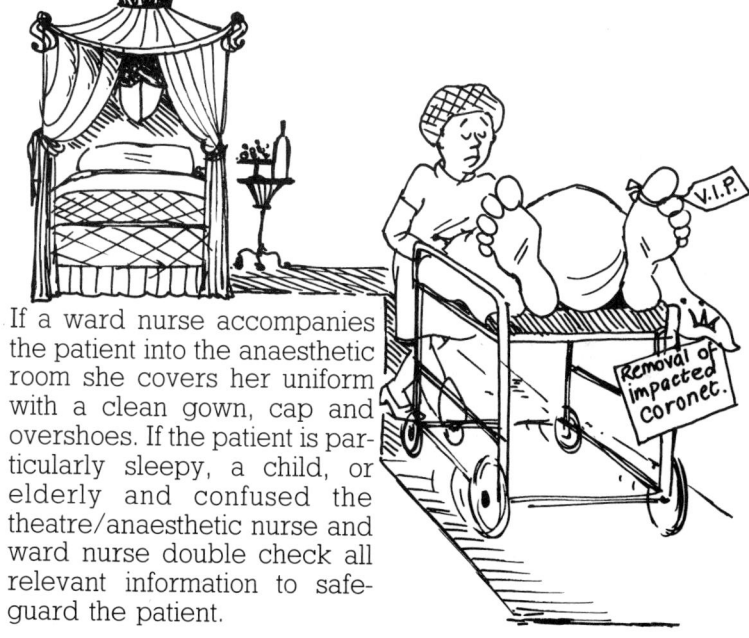

If a ward nurse accompanies the patient into the anaesthetic room she covers her uniform with a clean gown, cap and overshoes. If the patient is particularly sleepy, a child, or elderly and confused the theatre/anaesthetic nurse and ward nurse double check all relevant information to safeguard the patient.

3. ANAESTHETIC ROOM

Preparation before the patient arrives is important to allay anxieties.

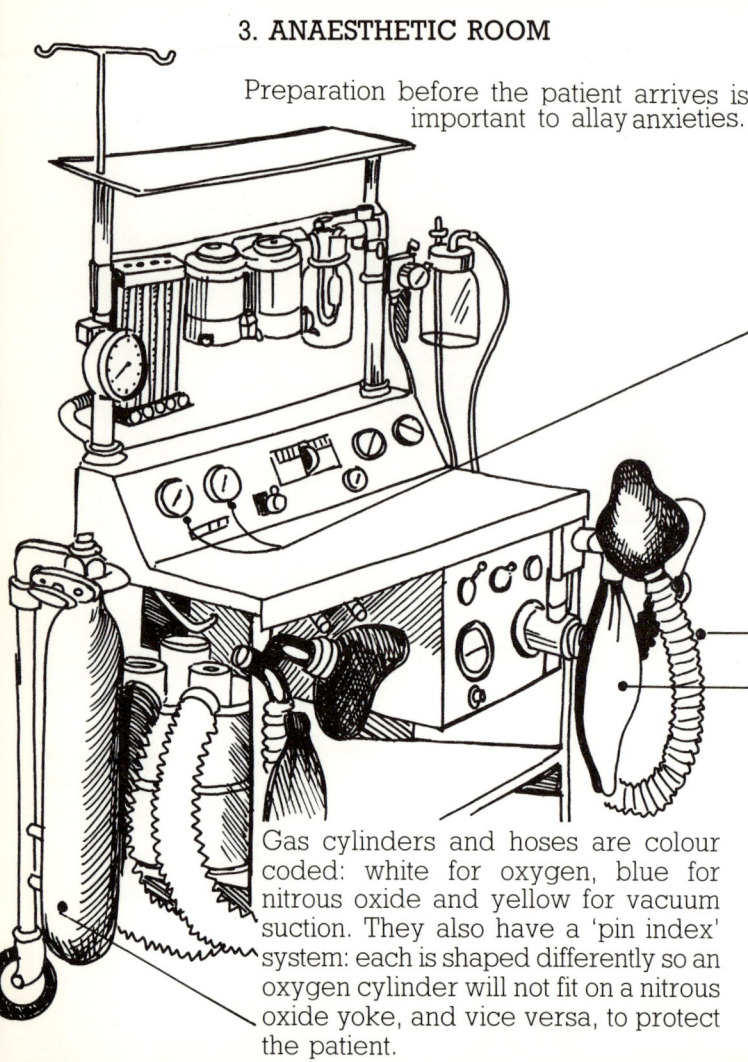

Gas cylinders and hoses are colour coded: white for oxygen, blue for nitrous oxide and yellow for vacuum suction. They also have a 'pin index' system: each is shaped differently so an oxygen cylinder will not fit on a nitrous oxide yoke, and vice versa, to protect the patient.

NURSE DUTIES: CHECKING

The alarm systems of the piped and cylinder oxygen and nitrous oxide must be checked. When the oxygen pressure drops an alarm sounds to prevent the patient from receiving only nitrous oxide. The main oxygen and nitrous oxide hoses are plugged in and the quantity of gas in the cylinders checked so that they are ready if the main hoses have to be disconnected.

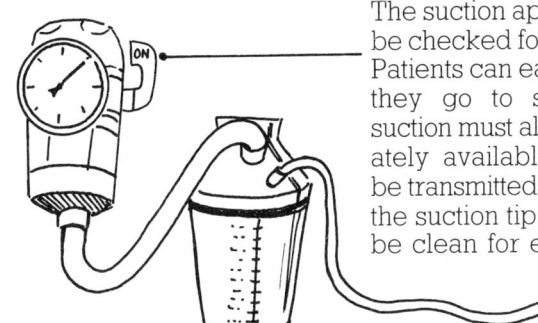

The suction apparatus needs to be checked for vacuum power. Patients can easily vomit just as they go to sleep, therefore suction must always be immediately available. Hepatitis can be transmitted through saliva so the suction tip and tubing must be clean for each patient.

Check the elephant tubing and rebreathing bag for leaks. Ensure that the anaesthetic machine has a selection of syringes and needles, a container for the disposal of sharps and a rubbish bag.

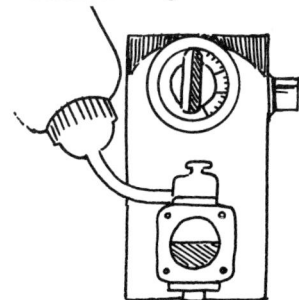

Then check that there is sufficient level of inhalational anaesthetic agents in the vaporisers (e.g. halothane). To protect the patient, modern vaporisers also have a system of special bottle tops so that halothane cannot be poured into enflurane vaporisers, etc.

Check the soda lime; if the colour has altered it will need changing.

EQUIPMENT

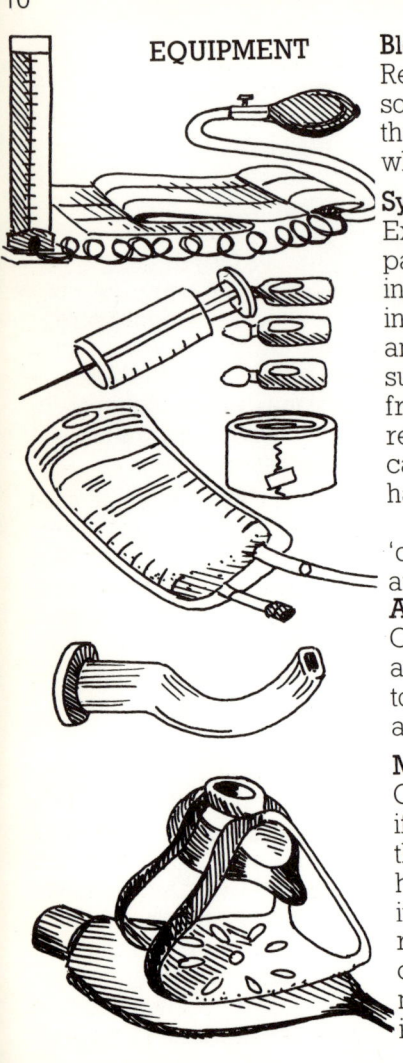

Blood pressure cuff
Record the blood pressure soon after the patient arrives as this gives a base line from which to assess later pressures.

Syringes, needles and tape
Except for small children all patients have an intravenous induction. Make sure that the induction drug (thiopentone) and muscle relaxants (curare, succinylcholine) are brought from the refrigerator and ready. Often an indwelling cannula is left in the vein so have tape ready.

Prepare an intravenous (IV) 'drip' solution according to the anaesthetist's choice.

Airway
Once the patient is asleep an airway is needed to keep the tongue out of the way. Select an appropriate size for the patient.

Mask and bag
Choose an appropriate size and if the mask is to be used throughout the operation then a harness will be needed to hold it on. The elephant tubing and rebreathing bag can be changed between patients to minimise respiratory cross-infection.

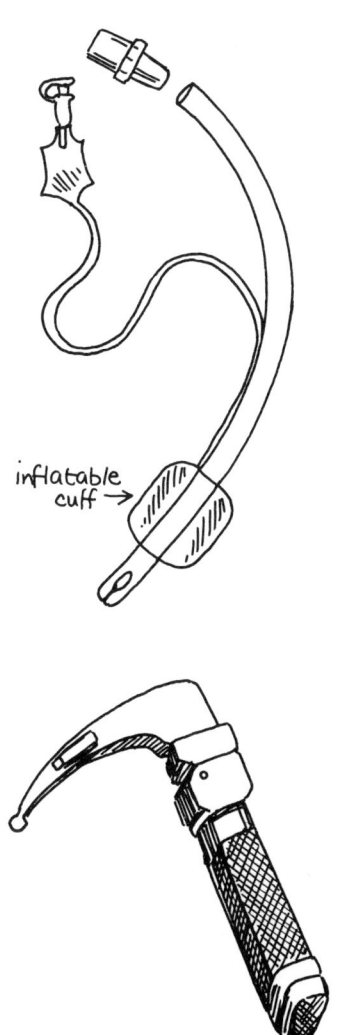

inflatable cuff →

Intubation equipment

An endotracheal tube may be required for many procedures. For example, if the surgeon needs access to the face, head and neck; if the procedure is major and the anaesthetist needs to deliver an accurate volume and concentration of anaesthetic; if the operation is long and holding a mask is impracticable; in chest and abdominal surgery where muscular relaxation is required which would inhibit breathing and a ventilator machine must take over. Some procedures, particularly on the cervix and anus, cause such stimulation that the patient may have a respiratory arrest and if intubated can be ventilated easily.

Laryngoscope

This is needed in order to visualise the vocal chords. Test the bulb to make sure it is screwed in tightly and not likely to fall into the patient's mouth, and check that the batteries give a bright light. Have a spare laryngoscope ready. Choose a laryngoscope blade of suitable size for the patient.

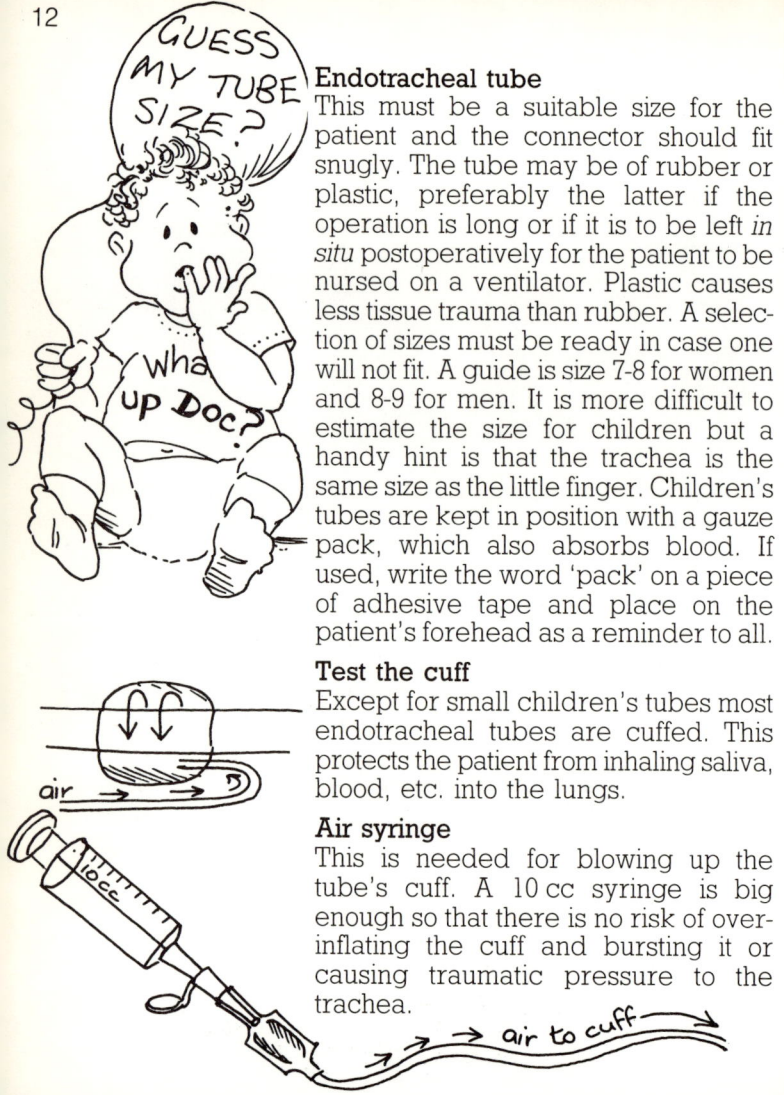

Endotracheal tube
This must be a suitable size for the patient and the connector should fit snugly. The tube may be of rubber or plastic, preferably the latter if the operation is long or if it is to be left *in situ* postoperatively for the patient to be nursed on a ventilator. Plastic causes less tissue trauma than rubber. A selection of sizes must be ready in case one will not fit. A guide is size 7-8 for women and 8-9 for men. It is more difficult to estimate the size for children but a handy hint is that the trachea is the same size as the little finger. Children's tubes are kept in position with a gauze pack, which also absorbs blood. If used, write the word 'pack' on a piece of adhesive tape and place on the patient's forehead as a reminder to all.

Test the cuff
Except for small children's tubes most endotracheal tubes are cuffed. This protects the patient from inhaling saliva, blood, etc. into the lungs.

Air syringe
This is needed for blowing up the tube's cuff. A 10 cc syringe is big enough so that there is no risk of over-inflating the cuff and bursting it or causing traumatic pressure to the trachea.

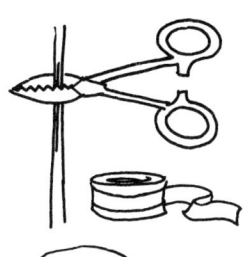

Clamp for cuff
This is to prevent air leaking out.

Tie or tape
This holds the tube in position. An airway is taped in as well to prevent the patient's teeth from squeezing or puncturing the tube.

Ointment or tape for the eyes
This is to protect the patient's cornea from drying or being damaged by drapes, blood, etc.

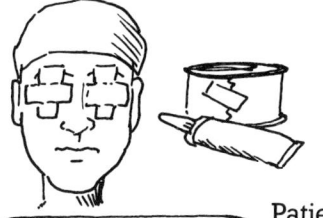

Patient monitoring devices
The following devices are required:

(1) An electrocardiogram (ECG) or pulse monitor.

(2) A blood pressure cuff or arterial line, for which you need (a) arm board and sandbag or IV bag to position the wrist, (b) alcohol swab for skin preparation, (c) cannula, (d) the heparinised 'flush' solution with connecting tubing and three-way taps, (e) transducer.

(3) A central venous pressure (CVP) line.

(4) Temperature probes.

(5) Urinary catheter and bag.

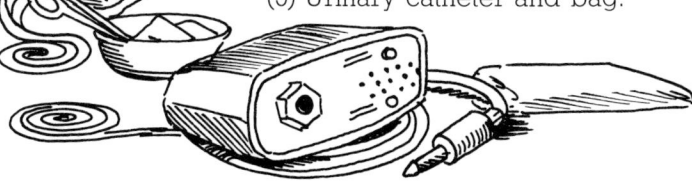

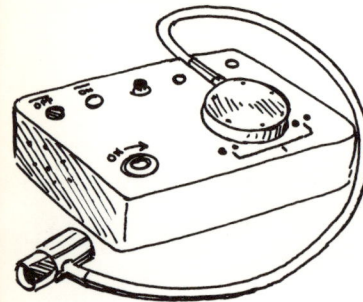

Equipment monitoring devices
Oxygen and ventilator pressure monitors are required. Switch on the ECG monitor alarms and set them approximately 20 beats above and below the patient's rate. Connect the scavenging system for exhaust gases to prevent pollution.

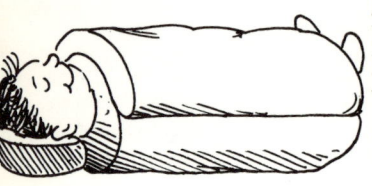

Extras
Hot water blanket, 'space blanket' (the foil reflects back the patient's heat) or fan to cool patient and/or staff in hot climates.

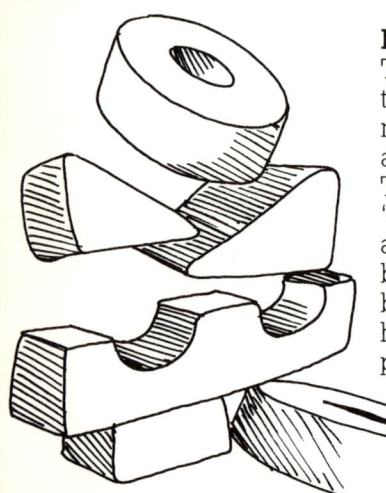

Positioning pads
These are to protect the patient's pressure areas and maintain the patient securely in a suitable position for surgery. These pads would include a 'doughnut' for the head and arm supports to protect the brachial nerve. Also a foam block would keep the patient's heels and calves off the bed to prevent deep vein thrombosis.

For back surgery, pillows are needed under the chest and hips to allow free abdominal movement for breathing. This also prevents a rise in venous pressure which may cause increased oozing in the surgical site.

Lithotomy poles should be padded. Similarly, any support pole for hip, kidney or chest surgery should be padded to protect the patient from pressure. Should there be an electrical fault with the diathermy the padding protects the patient's skin from a metal burn.

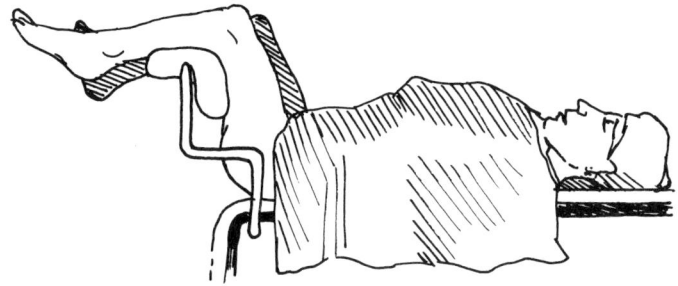

> The anaesthetic room is now ready. Obviously you would only select from this list equipment appropriate for the operation but an endotracheal tube should always be available for a patient just in case of difficulty or collapse.

PATIENT IN ANAESTHETIC ROOM

The anaesthetic nurse welcomes the patient warmly and asks the full name. This is verified with the name band on the wrist and the hospital notes. The hospital number is also checked. The accompanying nurse is asked for any special information about the patient such as the presence of an artificial eye or limb, and any handicap, e.g. deaf (take your mask down so that the patient can lip read!), paralysed, etc.

> The nurse must ask the patient if anything has been eaten or drunk within the past 4-6 hours (to avoid inhalation of stomach contents).
>
> She must then ask about any allergies or any medications being taken (check with drug chart) to avoid adverse interaction with anaesthetic agents. The presence of false teeth or crowns (to prevent inhalation or damage of plate) must be checked. Check that the patient's bladder has been emptied; this is particularly important prior to abdominal surgery.

Alert the anaesthetist to any information you have gained from the patient. The patient's pulse and blood pressure are recorded. It is essential that *'the patient is never left alone'*. If the mother has accompanied a small child find a book she can read to him. For adults and children alike the atmosphere should be calm, quiet and restful. Premedication often accentuates hearing so loud noises must be avoided. Take these few minutes to establish a rapport with the patient, who will shortly entrust you with his/her total care. Once the patient is asleep you become his/her sole representative; you should ensure that the patient is neither cold nor has a limb uncomfortably positioned. Due consideration should always be given for the patient's modesty and religious beliefs.

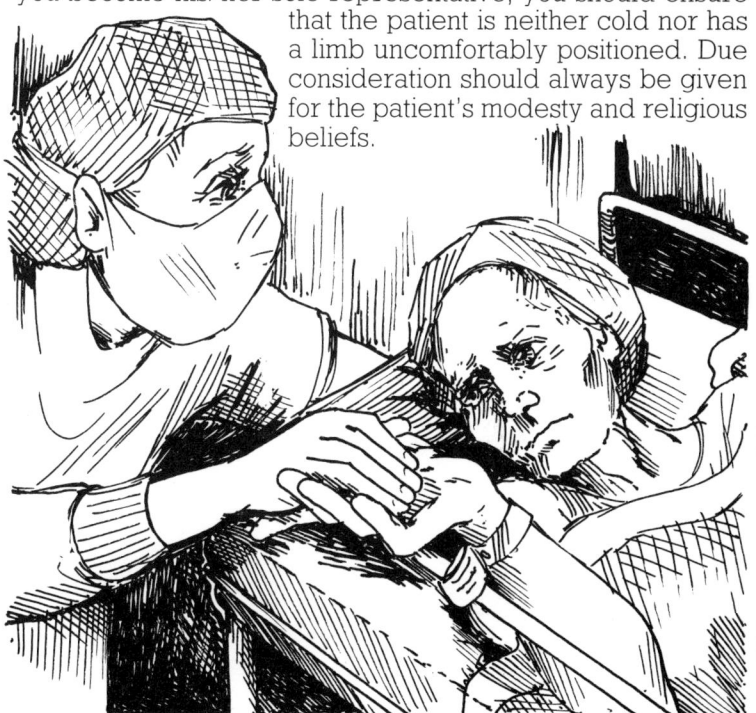

PATIENT ANAESTHESIA

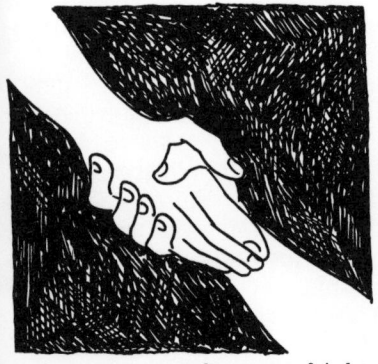

The anaesthetist has checked the equipment and the drugs he is to use. From this moment it is essential to stand beside the patient and help the anaesthetist. For reassurance, hold the patient's hand and say something positive like 'relax, you're among friends' or 'dream of good weather' or 'enjoy your sleep'. Suddenly losing consciousness can be very frightening to a patient so be there as a reassuring presence. You are also available to hold the patient's arms if they slip or to use suction if the patient vomits. The sense of hearing is the last to go so be careful about what is said in the anaesthetic room. Support the jaw to maintain the patient's airway. If an oro-pharyngeal airway is used, moisten or grease it lightly, since the tongue is dry and the airway may not slide in easily. If a relaxant has been given the anaesthetist will need to apply the face mask and insufflate the lungs for a minute using pure oxygen. Then pass the laryngoscope to the anaesthetist so that the vocal chords can be visualised. Pass him the lubricated endo-tracheal tube and help by holding back the patient's top lip and applying gentle cricoid pressure (just below the Adam's apple). If the patient has consumed food or fluid recently then firm cricoid pressure must be applied immediately he/she

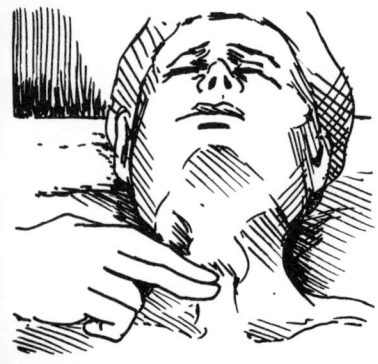

goes to sleep and not released until the cuff is inflated. The aim is to compress the oesophagus beneath the tracheal cartilage so no vomitus can be inhaled. This simple manoeuvre can be life saving. Ask the anaesthetist to show you how it is done before an emergency arises.

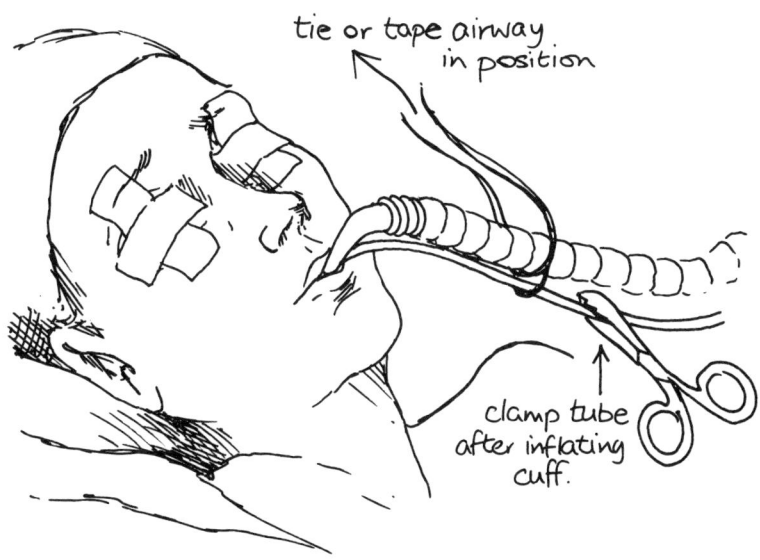

Once the tube is in position blow up the cuff gently until no air leaks from around it, then apply the clamp. Tape or tie the tube and airway in position. Care for the eyes. The anaesthetist will tell you what monitoring devices he wants each patient to have. *Ask* the anaesthetist before you move the patient or do anything further.

DRUGS USED IN ANAESTHESIA
This is a very big subject. Bear in mind that this book is just a 'thumbnail sketch'; for greater detail and understanding never be too over-awed to ask an anaesthetist. Choose your moment though! If in doubt precede your questions by 'is this a convenient time to ask?'.

Drugs fall into six main categories: premedication, induction agents, maintenance, narcotics, relaxants and reversants.

Premedication
This is to relax the patient and allay anxieties. (Remember that good preoperative teaching and reassuring nursing care is better than a larger dose of a drug.) Also given is an agent to dry mouth secretions to avoid inhalation of saliva. The relaxing part of the premedication may start the previous night with sedation. The patient may be given an oral premedication such as diazepam or lorazepam in the early morning or just an intramuscular (IM) injection of pethidine or papeveretum, for example. This narcotic also reduces the amount of induction agent needed. The anaesthetist must be alerted if the premedication has not been given or if it was given very shortly before the patient's arrival in theatre, since in this event the premedication could have its maximum effect once the patient is asleep and the blood pressure could then drop suddenly. If not given or given considerably longer than one hour preoperation, the anaesthetist can make appropriate adjustments to his drug dosages.

Atropine and scopolamine are the commonest mouth-drying agents. Atropine also affects the patient's eye focus and the tachycardia it gives is a beneficial side effect as thiopentone can cause bradycardia. The patient may need reassuring about eyes and heart rate because of these effects.

Induction agents
The commonest way to induce sleep is by using thiopentone. Other short-acting barbiturates may be used if, for example,

the patient is going home the same day. Ketamine, although rarely used (because of the hallucinations it gives), is particularly useful for burn patients. Once induced with Ketamine the patient can cough and swallow and maintain blood pressure well without much intervention, and this is considerably better than being subjected to frequent general anaesthetics for changes of dressings.

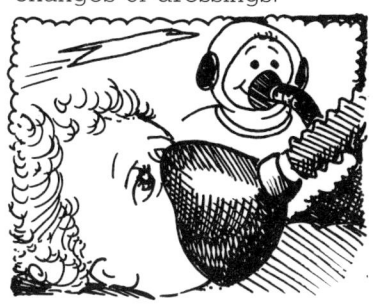

Small children are induced using the face mask with oxygen and adding increasing concentrations of nitrous oxide and halothane. Encourage a child by talking positively about 'blow up the balloon' (the re-breathing bag) or 'pretend the mask is like one worn by a pilot in a plane'.

Maintenance of anaesthesia
Commonly this is by using nitrous oxide which is both anaesthetic and analgesic. Another volatile gas such as halothane or enflurane can be added.

Narcotics
We now have oxygen plus nitrous oxide plus inhalational agent. To this can be added small incremental doses of a narcotic to keep the patient pain free. Physiologically the patient may feel pain, with changes in blood pressure and pulse indicating stress, but the patient is not mentally aware of pain. Common narcotics used are pethidine, morphine or fentanyl. This last drug is enjoying popularity as it is very potent, lasts up to an hour and does not affect the pupil reactions, which is important in neurosurgery. The effects are cumulative so decreasing quantities are needed. Everything given is to ensure that the patient has adequate anaesthesia and analgesia without being overwhelmed with drugs.

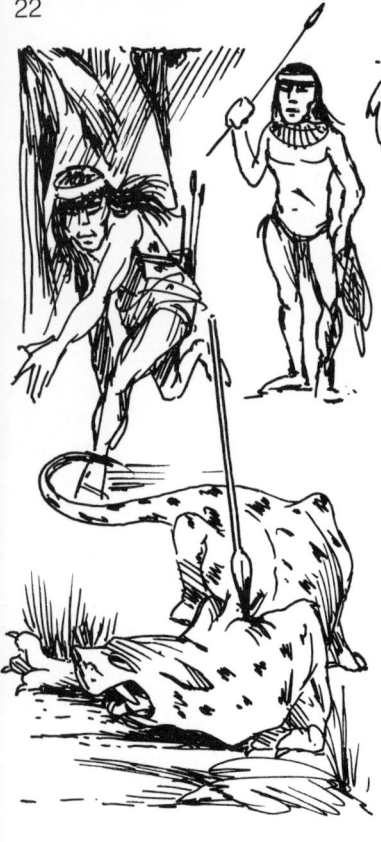

Relaxants

No matter how deeply asleep someone is, to attempt to pass an endotracheal tube would cause coughing and wretching. So the anaesthetist needs to give a muscle relaxant to temporarily paralyse the patient's muscles. There are two types of relaxant, the curare group (e.g. tubocurarine and pancuronium) and the depolarising drugs (e.g. suxamethonium and succinylcholine). Curare has been known for hundreds of years; the South American Indians used it on spears to paralyse animals prior to killing them. d-Tubocurarine (dtc) lasts approximately half an hour whereas pancuronium lasts nearly an hour.

If the anaesthetist just needs to intubate the patient and not maintain him on a ventilator then succinylcholine is used. This drug depolarises the muscle end-plate so that the nerve stimuli cannot get across. There is a transient stimulation so the patient twitches all over and then there is flaccid muscular relaxation which lasts for about three minutes. There is no antidote to succinylcholine; it is a matter of waiting for it to wear off.

Reversants

These are antagonists to the curare group of relaxants. The anaesthetist will have chosen the relaxant on the basis of the length of time of the operation. Even if the patient starts to breath again the drug must still be reversed to ensure none is left to cause respiratory difficulty later. Neostigmine is the drug used. It does cause a bradycardia so it is always given with atropine.

While neostigmine reverses the action of curare other stimulant drugs may be given to improve cardiac output or counteract the respiratory depressant effect of narcotics (e.g. naloxone).

REGIONAL ANAESTHESIA

The commonest regional anaesthetic is an epidural. The patient curls up on his side and the anaesthetist cleans the skin and inserts a needle into the epidural space at a suitable level from which there will be analgesia and muscle relaxation. Bupivacaine is commonly used as it lasts up to six hours. The advantage of an epidural anaesthetic is that the patient has no pain and has muscle relaxation which means no general anaesthetic is required. This is better for patients with lung problems. Epidural anaesthesia is excellent for caesarean sections, major abdominal and pelvic operations and hip replacement surgery. There is minimal blood loss and the epidural cannula can be left *in situ* (or put in during back operations like laminectomy) and topped up with further doses of bupivacaine for postoperative analgesia. It is essential that an IV is running during epidural anaesthesia in case of a profound drop in blood pressure. A brachial block is a regional anaesthetic for the arm, used, for example, in cases of plastic surgery to the tendons, etc.

LOCAL ANAESTHESIA

The commonest used is lignocaine. The ampoules or bottles must be kept and shown to the surgeon so he can verify the solution and strength he is using. Ensure there is minimum noise, preparations, counting equipment in theatre so as not to frighten the patient. If you drop something never say 'oops' but be positive and use 'there' instead.

It is essential that one nurse sits with the patient at all times, to distract with music, pictures or conversation and generally support the patient according to his/her needs. Patients undergoing eye surgery (often very old and frightened) are in particular need of quiet reassurance and should be reminded not to cough. (This raises intraocular pressure and can cause extrusion of vitreous humour, a disaster in cataract extraction.) Ensure the drapes are away from the patient's face, or if they must be closely applied, offer an oxygen mask so the patient can feel a flow of fresh air.

It is advisable that the patient stays in the operating theatre suite (a separate area of recovery) for a while after the procedure as the stress of even a minor procedure can greatly strain frail people (often chosen for local anaesthesia because of this frailty). Signs of local anaesthesia toxicity (confusion, garrulousness, twitching/convulsions) should be observed and reported.

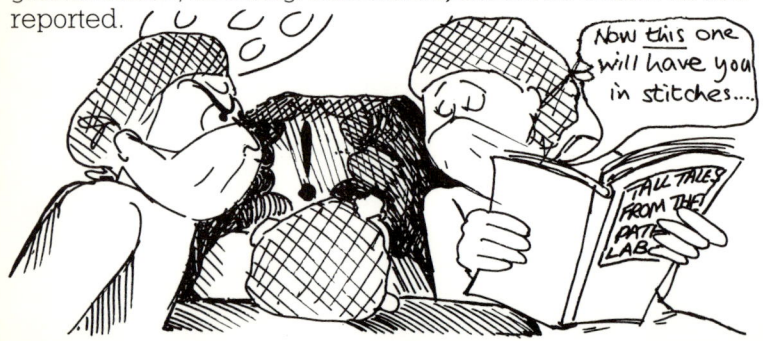

CARDIAC ARREST

If the patient arrests, don't panic, you have the key man of the resuscitation team right there! Sound the alarm to alert the other theatre staff. the anaesthetist will intubate and ventilate the patient while you do cardiac massage. He will establish an IV and the resuscitation drugs are kept in every anaesthetic room. The anaesthetist directs everyone to specific tasks. The surgeon will arrive and probably take over cardiac massage. You carry out your normal duties in an arrest: fetch the defibrillation trolley and plug it in, pass syringes and drugs as requested and make a note of event times.

4. PREPARATION OF THEATRE

CIRCULATING NURSE DUTIES

On first entering theatre the circulating nurse ('runner') should check the lights, including the operating lamps. Usually there is a positive pressure system of ventilation working so that fresh filtered air passes from ceiling to floor, is changed about 35 times every hour, and when a door is opened air flows out and no contaminated air is sucked in. Extremes of ventilation have been known from a glass enclosure with 300 air changes an hour, with body exhaust systems, to open doors and windows and care being taken that the pigeons don't get in! Temperature should be about 20°C (70°F) for everyone's comfort. Remember that the patient is under drapes and hot lights, although for babies theatre temperature is increased. Remember also that no one can work well if uncomfortably hot. Humidity is kept at a minimum of 50 percent to reduce the risk of static electricity sparks.

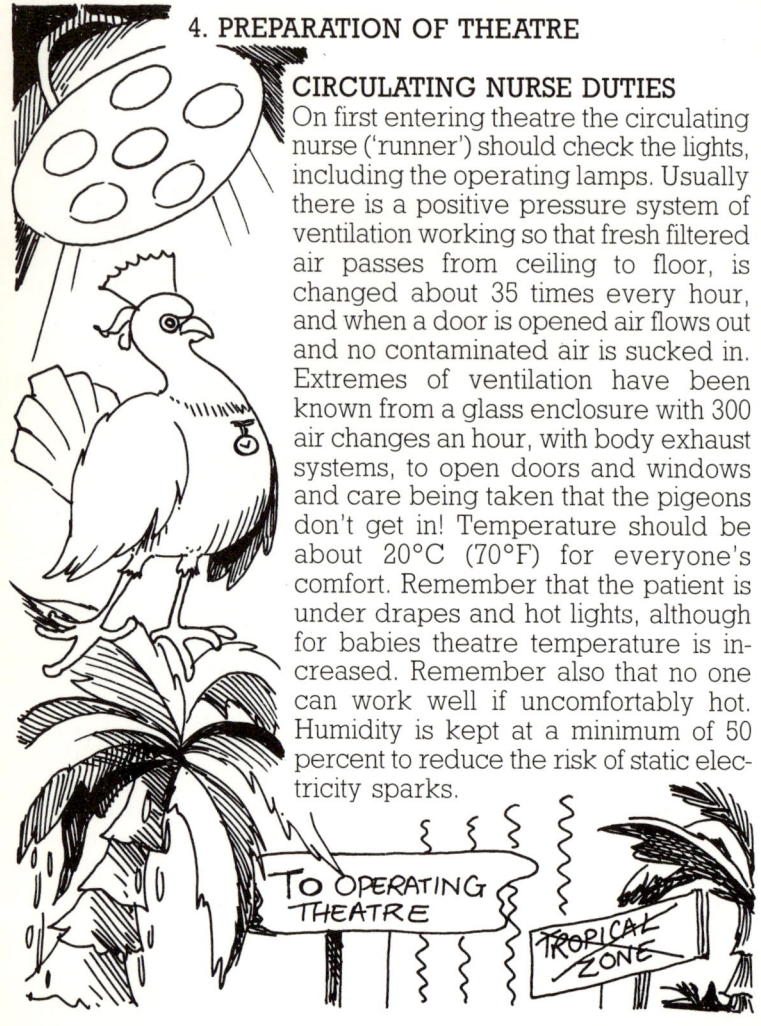

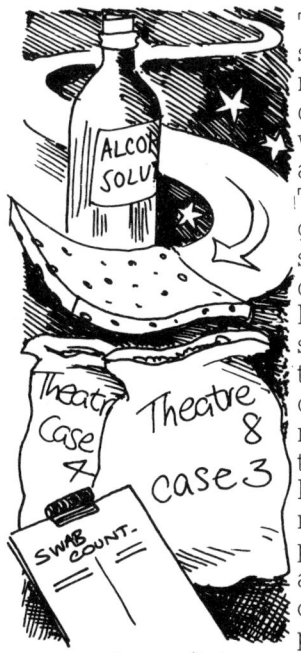

Theatres are cleaned thoroughly daily so there is no need to disturb the air more than is necessary at the beginning of a list. The surfaces are damp dusted with an alcohol solution. Fresh rubbish and laundry bags are labelled (e.g. Theatre 1 Case 1) so that if anything goes astray you know which bags to search! Write the patient's name and operation on the swab count board. Most theatres have a general supply shelf or trolley with preparation solutions, scalpel blades, sutures, dressings, etc. to minimise staff movement in and out of theatre. Make sure that this shelf is adequately stocked. Bring into theatre any extra equipment needed for this operation, e.g. compressed air cylinders, electrical apparatus, fibre optic light source, diathermy and suction machine, IV poles, etc.

To safeguard the patient no equipment should be used that has not been tested. Test the diathermy pedals and alarm system if the circuit breaks; test the suction jars for adequate vacuum; test that electrical equipment is plugged in and works. Check the temperature of the sterile water in the hot water cupboard; too hot could burn and too cold would send a patient into shock. Check that the operating table is locked in position, that any extras such as lithotomy poles are in the room ready and that the handle for tipping the table head down (in case the patient vomits) is there and you know how it works.

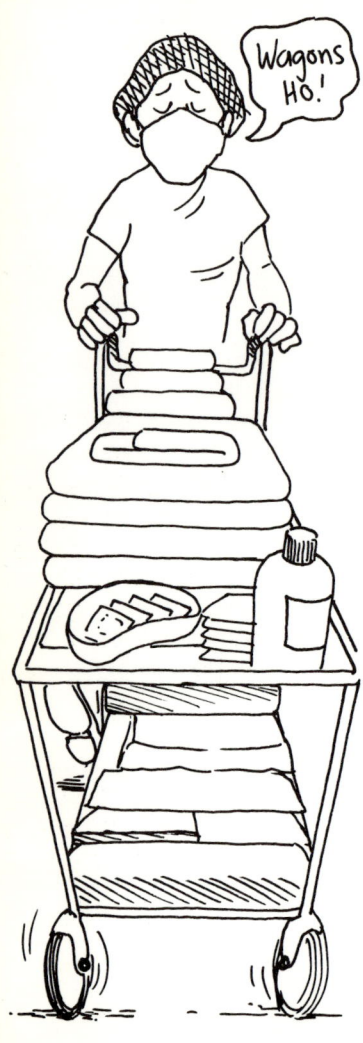

SCRUB NURSE DUTIES

Collect together all the instruments, extra swabs, sutures, drains, etc. that will be needed for the operation. Bundles and packets should be checked for sterility, i.e. that the autoclave tape has altered colour, that it is 'in date' (within the expiry date) and intact. *'If in doubt, throw it out.'*

Check with the surgeon's preference card for any extra items needed. It is important to try to think of any equipment that may be used during this case and have it ready to avoid subjecting the patient to long anaesthesia and open wound while someone goes to collect items. If the operation is a 'possible proceed' then collect all the materials for the second procedure also, to minimise change-over time. Save your circulating nurse's time by opening as many trays and packets as possible and your gown pack before scrubbing. The circulating nurse may have to double as an anaesthetic nurse and cannot help you simultaneously.

How to scrub

Make sure your cap and mask are comfortable and scratch your nose one more time! Scrubbing up is an important part of the surgical process and shouldn't be regarded as socialising around a bird bath. The aim is to clean the hands and forearms so that if a glove is punctured during surgery (even though the glove and instrument are discarded) there is minimal risk to the patient.

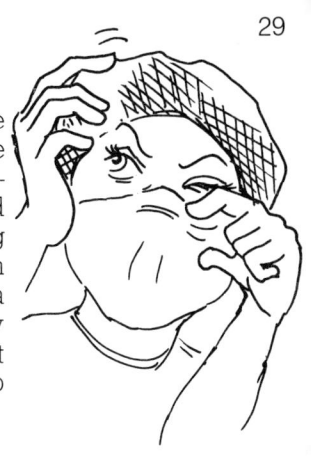

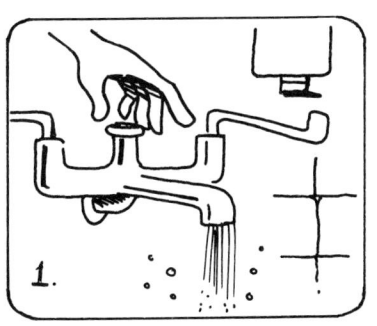

Select a comfortable water temperature and a scrub solution (often iodine or chlorhexidine). Wet the hands and forearms and wash them with the scrub solution. Either a disposable sponge/brush or a nailbrush may be used, as described below.

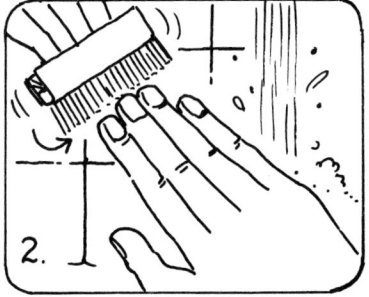

Disposable sponge/brush

Use the brush across the fingernails for 50 strokes for each hand. Turn the brush over, ensuring that it does not contact the palm of your hand.

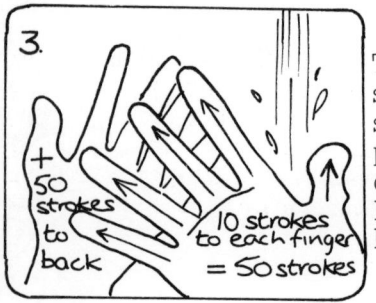

Then do 10 strokes along each side of each finger with the sponge. Do 50 strokes to the palm and 50 strokes to the back of the hand (= 10 to each finger). Repeat this process to the other hand.

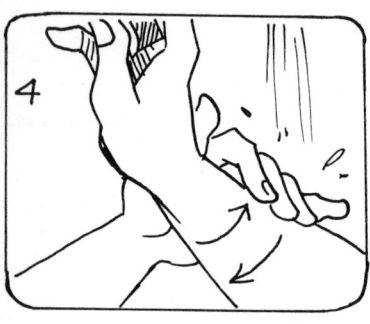

Then do 50 strokes to the front, sides and back of the wrist area. Repeat on the other arm.

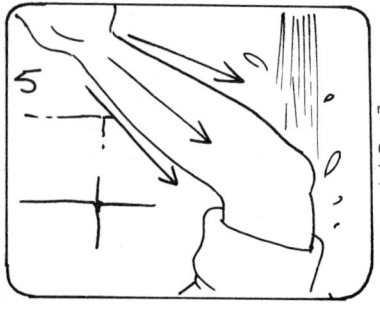

Then do 50 strokes to each side of the forearm to the elbow. Repeat the other side.

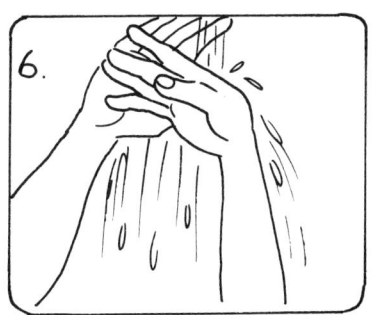

Rinse off, keeping the hands higher than the elbows to stop dirty water trickling back down over the hands. This only takes 3-5 minutes and you know that each hand is cleaned equally.

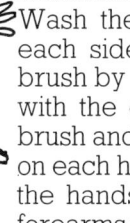

Nailbrush

Wash the forearms for 50 strokes to each side of each arm. Take a nailbrush by opening the brush dispenser with the elbow, apply solution to the brush and scrub the nails for 50 strokes on each hand. Discard the brush. Rinse the hands and forearms. Rewash the forearms with 50 strokes each arm and reapply solution to the hands and wash for 50 strokes to each finger, the palm and the back. Rinse off, taking care the hands are higher than the elbows. Be careful not to touch the taps, sink, etc. or you will have to start again. Your dress should not get wet either as this encourages bacterial growth which can permeate the gown and contaminate the patient. Drip off as much as possible in the sink. Theatre floors are 'lethal' when wet!

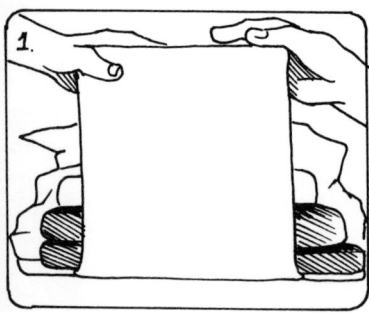

GOWNING AND GLOVING

Taking care no dirty water from the elbows trickles down on to the pack, open the inner gown wrap, take a towel and open it out. Dry the fingers, palm and back of one hand thoroughly.

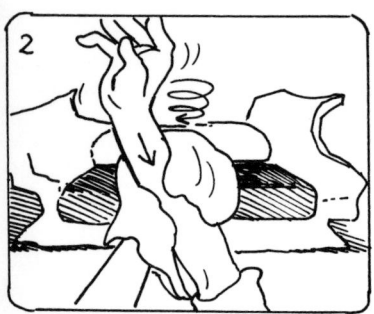

Protecting the other hand, with the towel grasp the wrist and corkscrew spiral down the arm, to dry it, ending at the elbow. Take a clean towel and repeat for the other hand and arm.

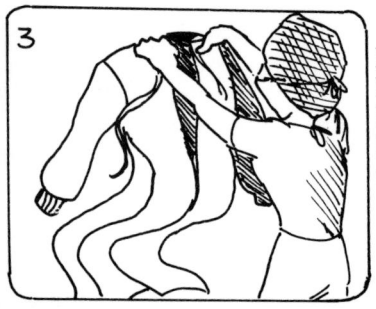

Pick up the gown and let the bottom unfold. Keep your hands on the inside and ensure the ties do not flap from the unsterile to sterile side.

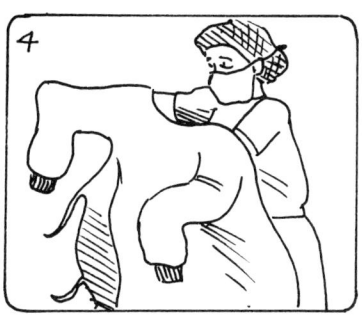

Open the gown and put your hands in the sleeves simultaneously. Keep your hands inside the sleeves.

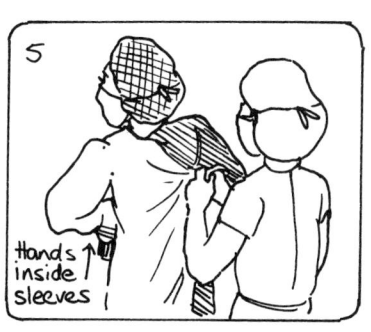

Let the circulating nurse pull the gown on you from behind and tie the tapes.

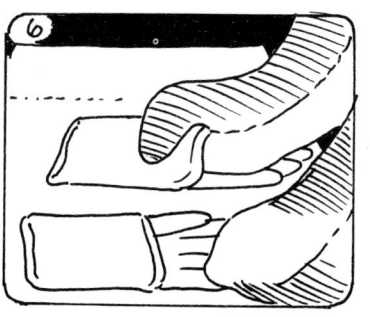

Take your gloves from the sterile packet opened by the circulating nurse. Open out the packet. Pick up one glove by its cuff.

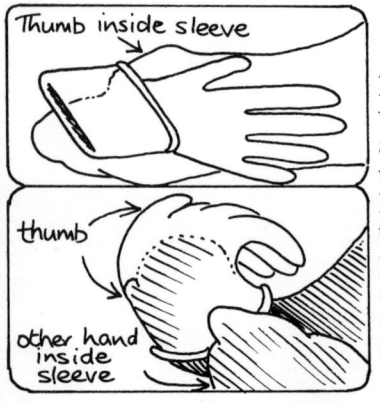

Lay it on the palm of your hand with the fingers pointing up the arm, with the thumb of the glove to your thumb inside the sleeve. Hold the cuff of the glove thumb to thumb. With the other hand pull the cuff over the sleeve and slide your fingers through and into the glove. Repeat with the other glove.

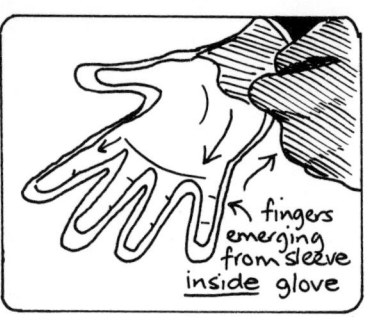

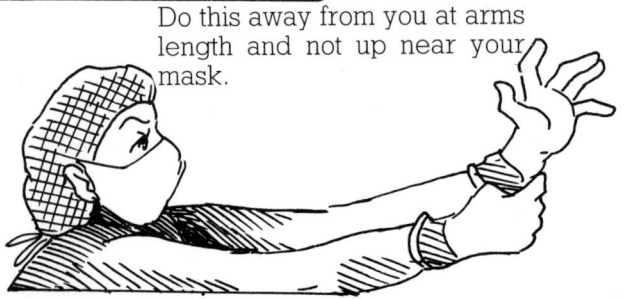

Do this away from you at arms length and not up near your mask.

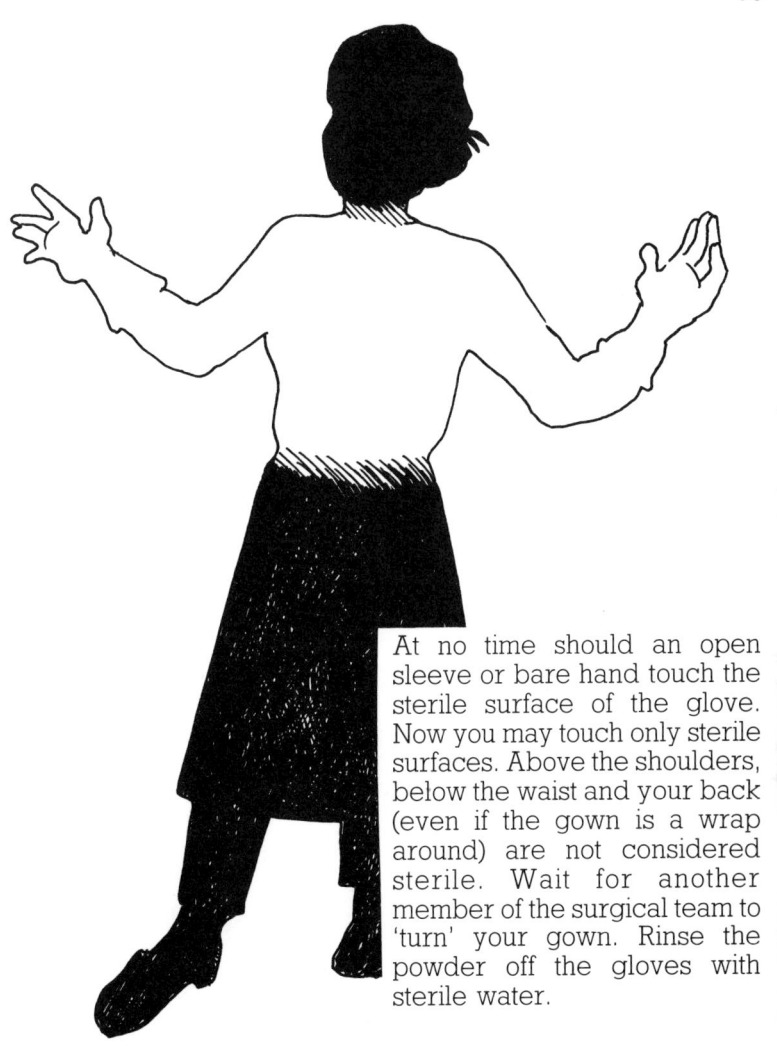

At no time should an open sleeve or bare hand touch the sterile surface of the glove. Now you may touch only sterile surfaces. Above the shoulders, below the waist and your back (even if the gown is a wrap around) are not considered sterile. Wait for another member of the surgical team to 'turn' your gown. Rinse the powder off the gloves with sterile water.

Setting up trolleys

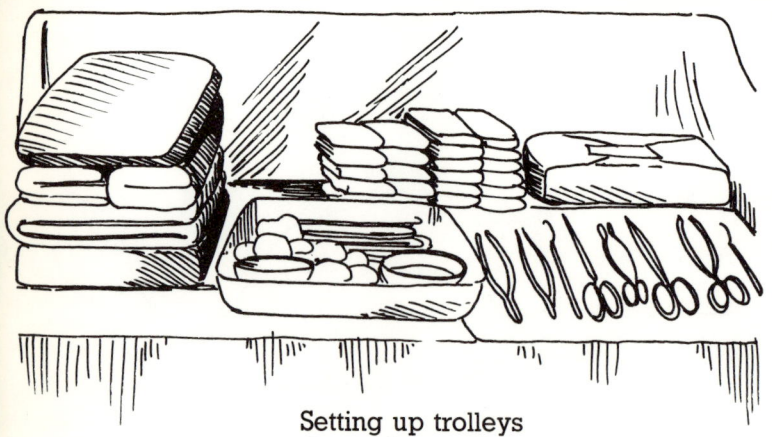

Open the sterile wraps towards you first, being sure to protect your gloves at all times from unsterile surfaces. Now you can stand close to the trolley with a sterile gown touching a sterile drape. As you pick up the patient drapes place them in the order you will use them (waterproof first, then a large sheet, two side sheets and a top sheet as a basic guide), thereby saving time and cutting down on unnecessary movement.

Skin preparation

This comes first so have the gallipot filled with the appropriate solution. Check the label and make sure the circulating nurse does not splash solution on the instruments. Put the skin preparation sponge holders easily available so that the surgeon can help himself if required.

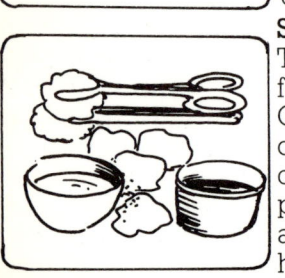

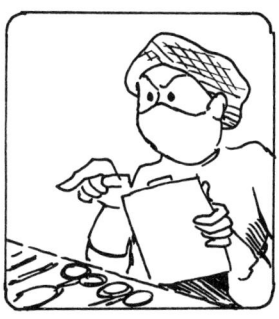

Count instruments
You are responsible for every item in use on the sterile field so make sure you know exactly what you have.

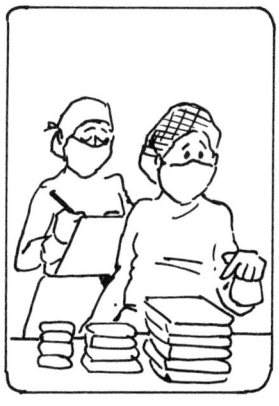

Count swabs
This must be done audibly with the circulating nurse and she must write it down immediately. When counting, separate each swab (so there is no risk of counting a fold) and make sure that both of you can see the X-ray detectable line. For abdominal swabs check that there is a tape as well as the X-ray detectable mark. Be conscientious in your count: patients depend on you to protect them.

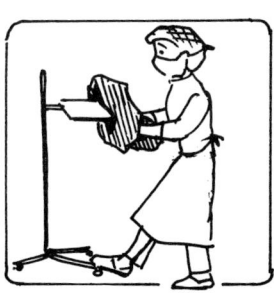

Cover the Mayo stand
Put your hands inside the Mayo drape cuff. Grasp the Mayo tray (with your foot on the bottom of the stand so it doesn't escape!) and slide the Mayo cover on. As it unfolds be sure it does not drop below waist level and become contaminated. Hold the end with your elbow at your waist as you slide the cover on.

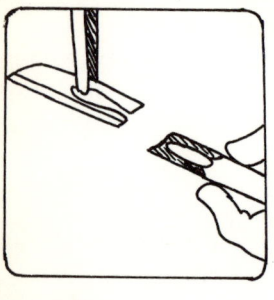

Scalpel blades

Take each blade from the circulating nurse and mount on the handle. Use an instrument to do this. At no time should the cutting edge of the scalpel blade come into contact with your glove. Slide the blade on the handle with the slopes of the blade and handle matching.

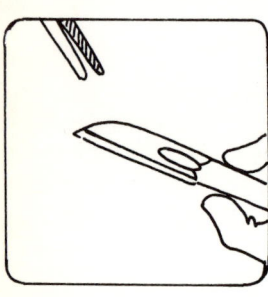

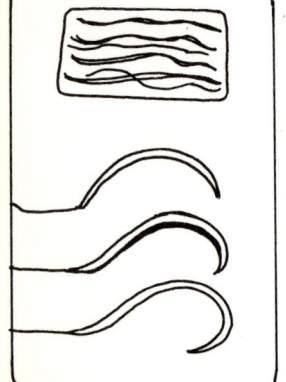

Sutures

Arrange these in order of use with the skin suture furthest away. Arrange ties in a separate place.

5. THE OPERATION

Once an operation begins, *nothing leaves theatre* without permission.

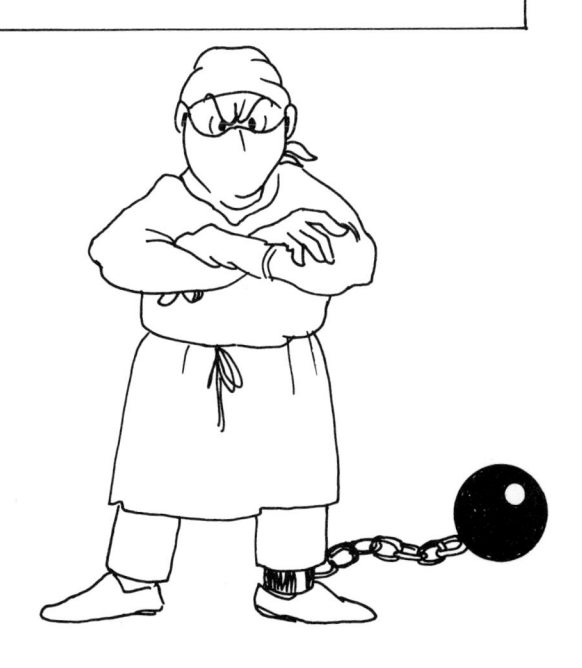

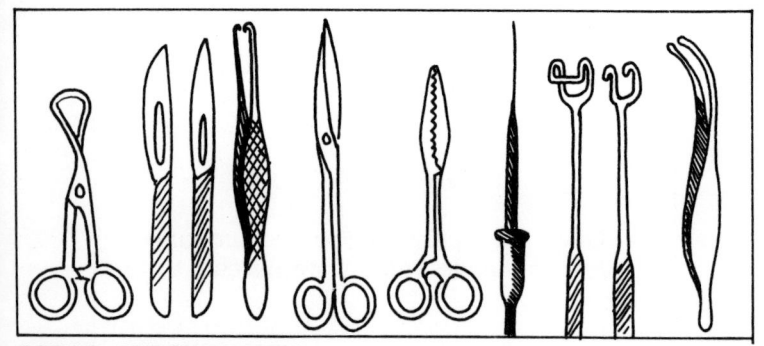

SCRUB NURSE DUTIES
The Mayo stand

Only the essential starting instruments need be placed on the Mayo tray. You read from left to right, so set up instruments in a similar logical way. Draping comes first so a few towel clips are needed (replace any unused clips on back table). Then the surgeon cuts, so skin knife is required, and beside that the inside knife. Toothed dissecting forceps are needed to hold the tissue while he cuts, and scissors next for further dissection. By now there's bleeding, so artery forceps will be needed. The diathermy active electrode (pencil or forceps) should be clipped to the drapes ready to seal bleeding points. Retractors will be required to hold tissue out of the way while dissection continues. These are placed above the other instruments. Next tissue holding forceps will be needed. Suction should be clipped up with the diathermy, and to prevent it sliding off the sterile area should be kept in the diathermy's quiver (holder). Swabs mounted on sponge holders may be needed now.

Clip suction-tube up beside the diathermy needle.

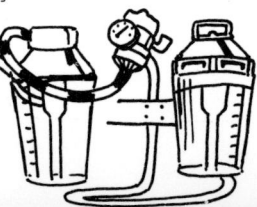

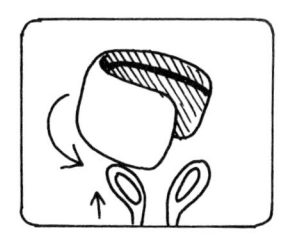

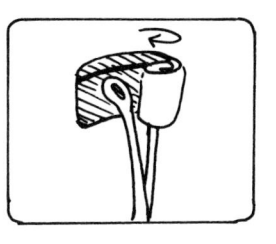

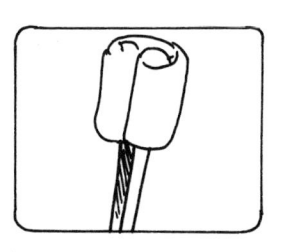

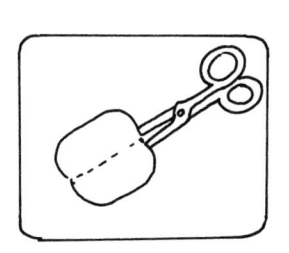

Mounting a swab on a sponge holder

Take a gauze swab and fold it in half with the X-ray detectable line inside (it can be harsh on patient's tissue). Place the open sponge holder in the middle and wrap over first one side and then the other. The tips of the sponge holder should not be visible so that they do not poke against the patient's tissues. When removing used swabs, touch (preferably with spare non-toothed dissecting forceps) only the base, and discard it, thereby minimising contact with the gloves.

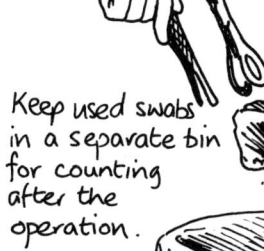

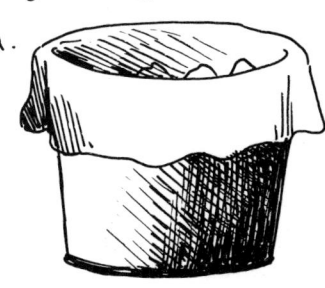

Keep used swabs in a separate bin for counting after the operation.

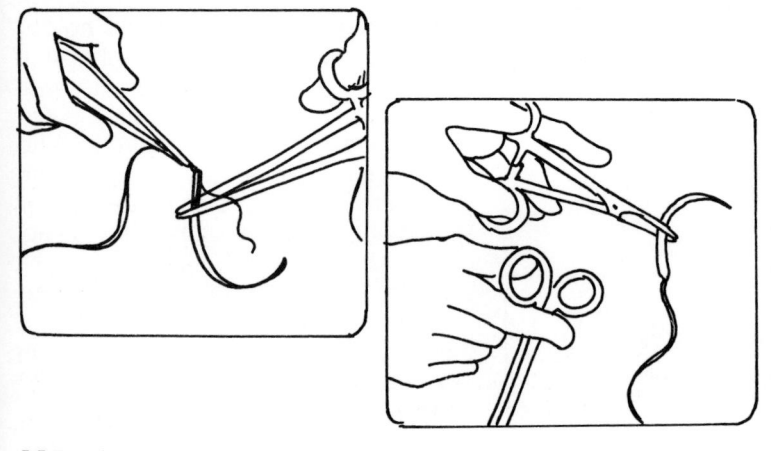

Mounting a suture

The tissue has been excised and a suture is required to start closure. Keep the needle holders down on your back table next to the sutures. To mount a suture open the packet *down and away* from you so there is no risk of the preservative solution splashing in your eyes. Tear the end off the packet and pull out the cardboard wrapper. Follow the suture makers' instructions! They tell you where to put your thumb and which piece of wrapper to lift. Hold the needle between the thumb and forefinger of the left hand so the tip is not touching your glove. Clip the needle holder on one third of the way from the end of the needle and at the tip of and at right angles to the holder. As you pull the cardboard wrapper off *(across* your set-up not above your shoulders *remember)* be sure not to touch the suture material especially if it is chromic catgut. The chromic acid comes off on your glove and reduces the quality of the suture. Hold the end of the suture gently until the surgeon has control of it. Whenever you hand up a suture also pass the assistant's scissors (kept with other scissors on the Mayo stand but handles opposite way up for quick siting).

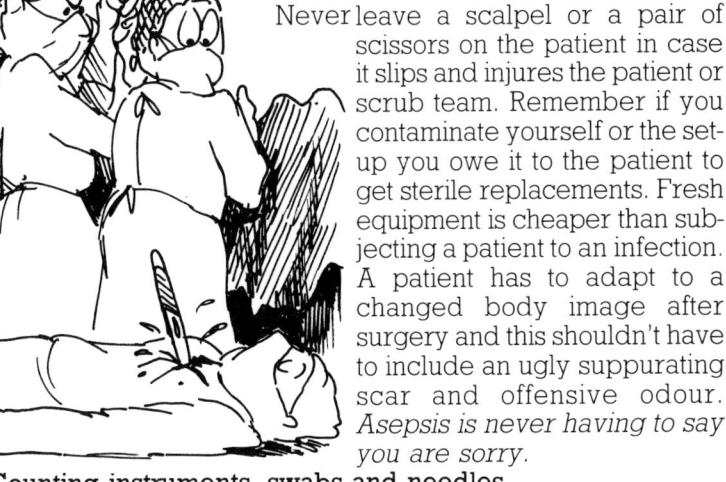

AT ALL TIMES KEEP ONE EYE ON THE WOUND!

Never leave a scalpel or a pair of scissors on the patient in case it slips and injures the patient or scrub team. Remember if you contaminate yourself or the set-up you owe it to the patient to get sterile replacements. Fresh equipment is cheaper than subjecting a patient to an infection. A patient has to adapt to a changed body image after surgery and this shouldn't have to include an ugly suppurating scar and offensive odour. *Asepsis is never having to say you are sorry.*

Counting instruments, swabs and needles

Once you have handed up a closure suture you must count your instruments, swabs and needles. This should be completed before the cavity is closed. Ultimately the surgeon is responsible if a swab is lost so he must allow reasonable time (rarely!) for a count to be done. Remember you are protecting the patient so do not hand up any further suture material until the count is complete. Inform the surgeon that the count is done and is correct. If it is not correct a re-count should be done, everything searched and an X-ray taken if necessary. If still not found the senior theatre nurse is informed and an incident report written at the end of the case. No matter how minor the procedure swabs are *always* counted; surgeons have a habit of doing a little bit more exploratory surgery.

A useful way of keeping track of the needles used is to stick them in their packet. Then at all times you know how many needles and what type of suture material is in use at any given time, and this speeds the count and disposal.

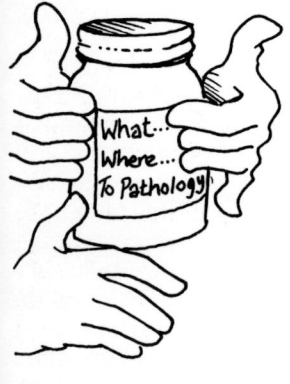

Care of specimen

Ask the surgeon if *any* tissue you receive is required as a specimen. Handle it very gently, with gloves or a swab and preferably not with an instrument. The pathologist has to view this piece under a microscope and toothed instruments damage and distort the tissue. As it is handed over to the circulating nurse (take care not to contaminate yourself on the specimen pot, or be splashed by its formalin) explain *what* it is and *where* it is from so she can label it properly.

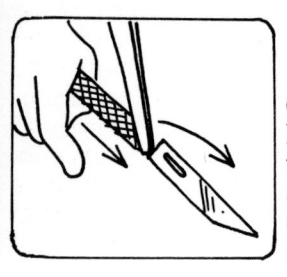

Clearing away equipment

Meanwhile the surgeon has sutured the wound closed and you repeat a count at skin closure. Obtain dressings and clear away your equipment. When removing scalpel blades use an instrument. Lift the heel of the blade pointing it *down and away* from you so there is no risk of it springing up and puncturing your eye. All sharps are disposed of together to prevent injury to nursing and ancillary staff.

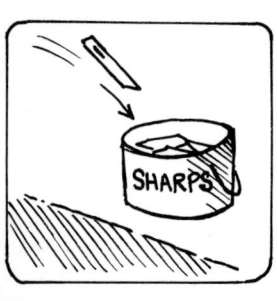

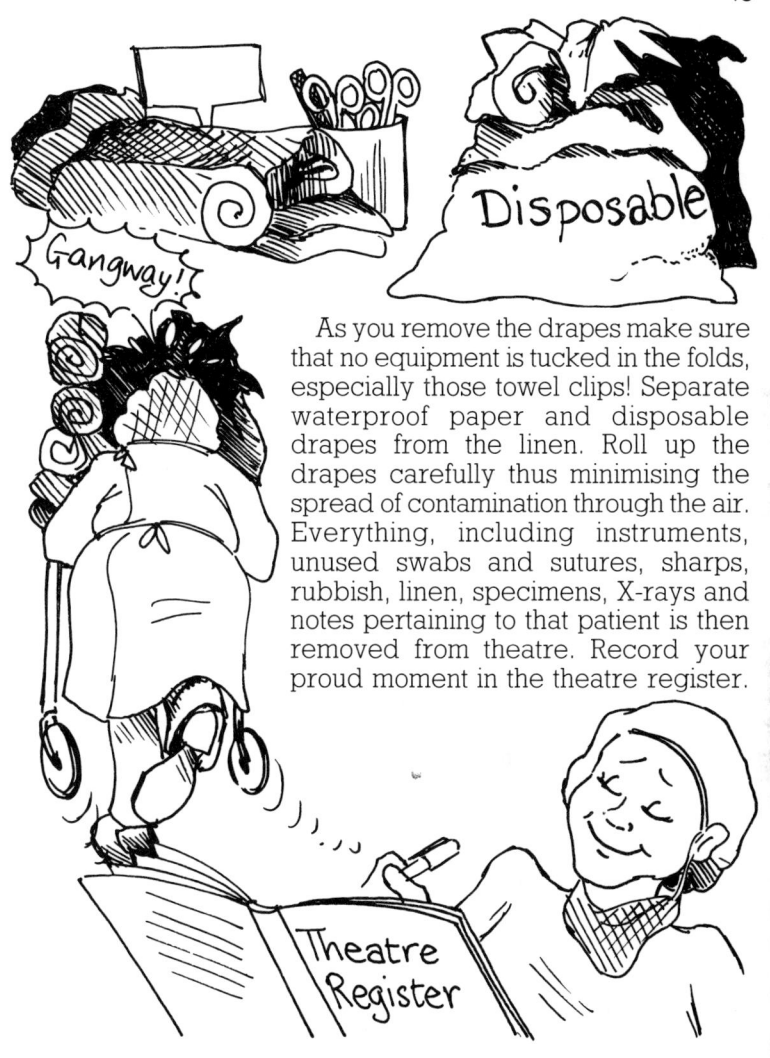

As you remove the drapes make sure that no equipment is tucked in the folds, especially those towel clips! Separate waterproof paper and disposable drapes from the linen. Roll up the drapes carefully thus minimising the spread of contamination through the air. Everything, including instruments, unused swabs and sutures, sharps, rubbish, linen, specimens, X-rays and notes pertaining to that patient is then removed from theatre. Record your proud moment in the theatre register.

CIRCULATING NURSE DUTIES

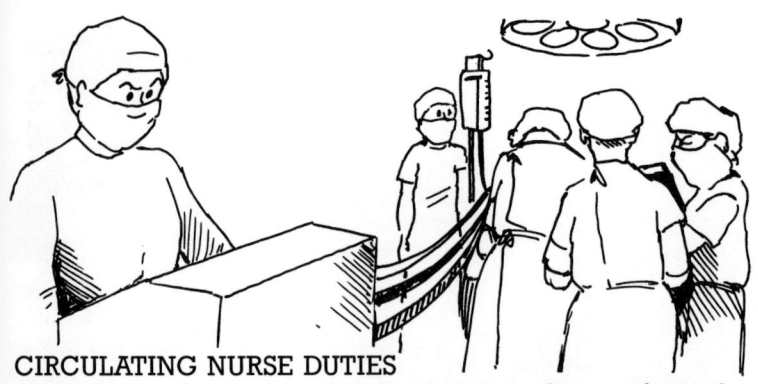

As soon as the patient is wheeled into theatre from the anaesthetic room help the anaesthetic nurse position the patient and get the anaesthetist settled. This is very important, particularly if (for example during neurosurgery) the anaesthetist will have limited access to the patient's head, the endotracheal tube, the IV site, etc. To protect the patient the anaesthetist must be sure all the connections are snug, IVs running and monitors working before the surgical team move in.

Remembering you are the patient's representative, check that the arms are well supported, that the patient isn't needlessly exposed, that pressure areas are guarded and that the patient is in a secure position, without joints or limbs uncomfortably over-extended or cramped. Be sure that the diathermy passive electric plate has good contact with the patient's skin, has no preparation solution on it and is properly connected so there is no risk of a burn to the patient.

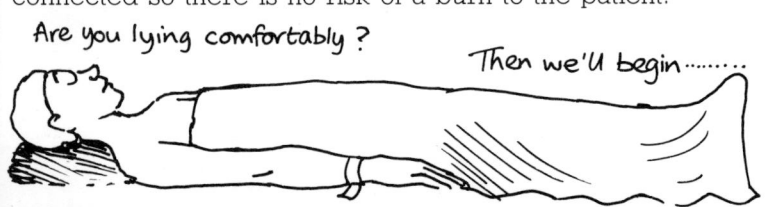

As the scrub nurse hands off the end of the active electrode diathermy lead attach it to the machine, ask which number of coagulation is required, turn it on and place the pedal at the surgeon's foot. Attach the suction to the vacuum bottle and turn on. Pour water into the scrub nurse's basin. Adjust the operating lamp over the wound if need be. Remain immediately available at all times; never leave the scrub nurse unless directed to do so. Anticipate the needs if more swabs or sutures are required.

Nothing leaves theatre once the case has started.

Swabs

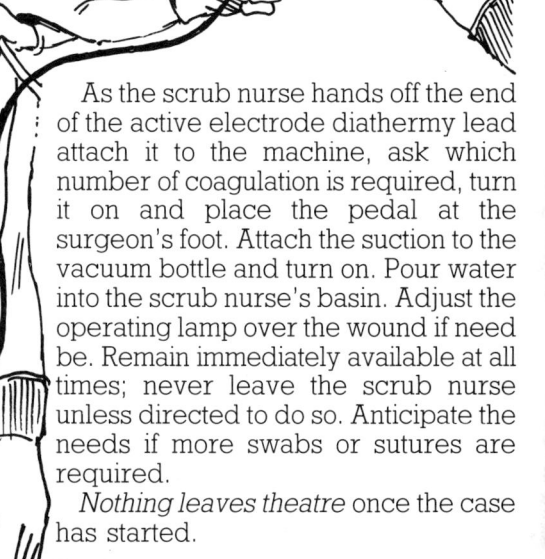

Use a sponge holder to pick up used swabs and hang them on the rack. *Never* pick up a bloody swab with your hands as you risk infection (hepatitis particularly) yourself and cross-infection to others if you then touch suture boxes, etc. which are used for everyone.

Specimens

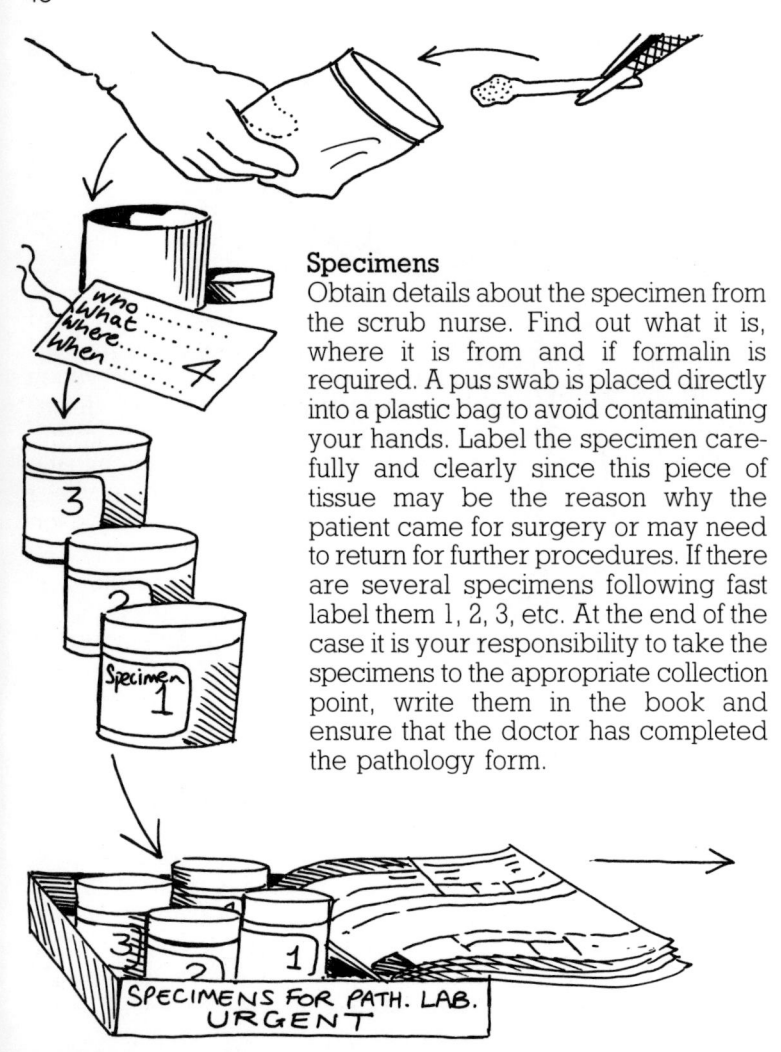

Obtain details about the specimen from the scrub nurse. Find out what it is, where it is from and if formalin is required. A pus swab is placed directly into a plastic bag to avoid contaminating your hands. Label the specimen carefully and clearly since this piece of tissue may be the reason why the patient came for surgery or may need to return for further procedures. If there are several specimens following fast label them 1, 2, 3, etc. At the end of the case it is your responsibility to take the specimens to the appropriate collection point, write them in the book and ensure that the doctor has completed the pathology form.

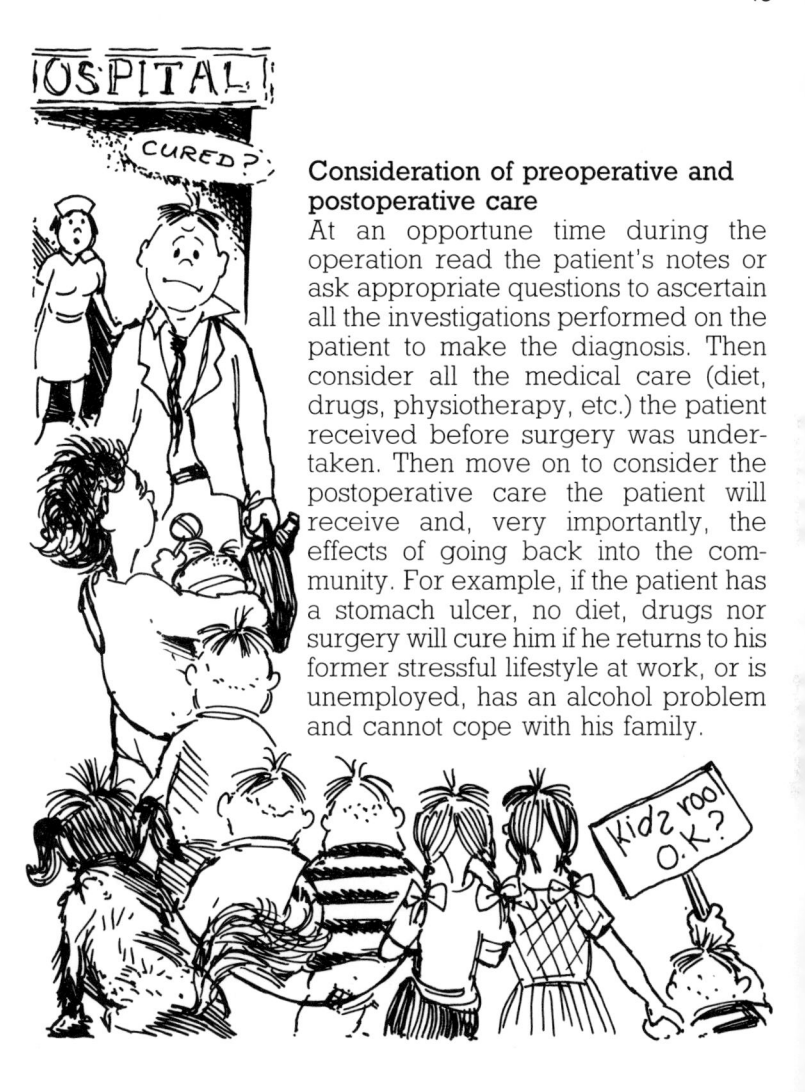

Consideration of preoperative and postoperative care

At an opportune time during the operation read the patient's notes or ask appropriate questions to ascertain all the investigations performed on the patient to make the diagnosis. Then consider all the medical care (diet, drugs, physiotherapy, etc.) the patient received before surgery was undertaken. Then move on to consider the postoperative care the patient will receive and, very importantly, the effects of going back into the community. For example, if the patient has a stomach ulcer, no diet, drugs nor surgery will cure him if he returns to his former stressful lifestyle at work, or is unemployed, has an alcohol problem and cannot cope with his family.

CARDIAC ARREST

If the patient has a cardiac arrest during the operation, don't panic, you have all the team there! Usually the anaesthetist will direct everyone. The surgeon commences cardiac massage while the anaesthetist intubates and ventilates the patient. One nurse must help the anaesthetist by collecting the defibrillation trolley and emergency drugs, pumping IVs, preparing syringes for drugs, recording times, etc. The other nurse assists the surgeon; this may entail relieving him of cardiac massage if, for example, the most important thing for him to be doing is controlling haemorrhage. Remember you can break scrub and sterile techniques at any time in this situation. If the patient survives, antibiotics can be given, but sterility is useless to a mortuary-bound patient. Once the patient has been resuscitated, gowns and gloves can be changed, drapes renewed, etc.

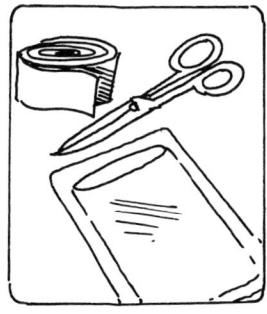

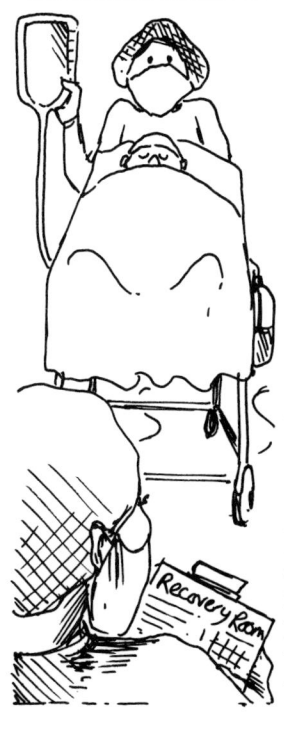

End of operation duties

At the end of the operation remember that it is a communal roll of dressing plaster so use clean scissors to cut it, not those from the surgical set. Neostigmine, the drug used to reverse curare form relaxants, contracts smooth muscle so get that colostomy bag on quickly!

The scrub nurse deals with the soiled drapes as she is protected by her gown and gloves. You concentrate on assisting the anaesthetist: suction is required to clear the patient's mouth prior to extubation, monitoring equipment may need to be removed, the eye tapes need to be removed and a nurse accompanies the patient and anaesthetist to the recovery room. Hand over your patient to the recovery nurse, stating the patient's name, the operative procedure performed, any drains or equipment *in situ*. Return to theatre and assist in disposing of the rubbish from the previous case, clean the swab board, wash your hands and start setting up for the next case.

At the end of the day the theatre must be cleaned. Hot soapy water is best. Start at the lights, work down methodically, moving round the room cleaning furniture and ending with the stools and waste buckets. Use disposable cloths, with spirit for glass and metal.

6. RECOVERY ROOM

PREPARATION

At the beginning of first shift (or some quiet period of the evening/night), when no patients are in the vicinity, test the cardiac arrest alarm bells. Every patient area has oxygen and suction, both of which must be tested. Routine equipment such as blood pressure cuffs, plasters, dressings, etc. must be checked for adequate supplies. The recovery room has its own resuscitation trolley. A check must be made for the presence of all the requirements for intubation: drugs, IVs, bottles, needles, tape, etc. This equipment is functionally checked the same as in an anaesthetic room.

Ensure that there are adequate supplies of tissues and vomit bowls, wash cloths and basins, IV bottles/bags and those old familiar friends — bedpans and bottles!

Check the cardiac arrest alarm bells!

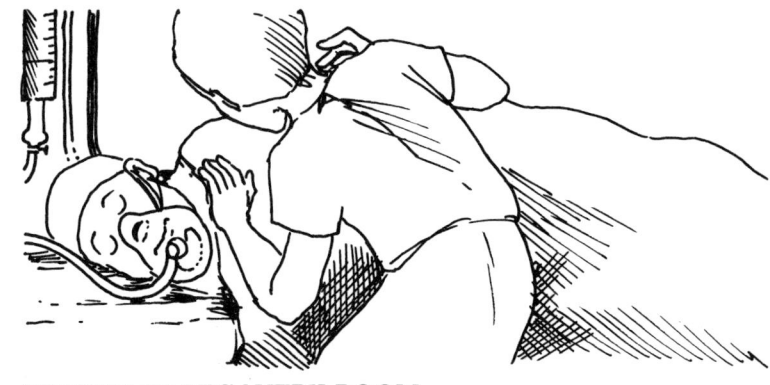

PATIENT IN RECOVERY ROOM

As soon as the patient arrives the recovery room nurse learns the patient's name and the operative procedure that has been performed. The anaesthetist will inform you of any special observations and treatment needed. As with any unconscious patient the first priority is to maintain a clear airway. The patient may need to be positioned on the right or left side after ear, nose and throat procedures and suction should be readily available for blood, vomit, mucus, etc. Oxygen is given routinely. Nitrous oxide given as part of the general anaesthesia is exhaled and the patient can breathe greater concentrations with shallow respiration. Oxygen 'blows away' the exhaled gases and assists a rapid recovery.

Hopefully, part of the preoperative teaching mentioned the patient waking up with an oxygen mask on and probably an IV going. To many lay people these are signs of critical illness and they are frightened. Reassure the patient that the mask is just 'fresh air' and the IV is replacing their missed morning tea.

> Normal Service *will* be resumed as soon as possible

Regular observations (at least every 15 minutes) are made of the patient's pulse, blood pressure and respiration. These are noted and compared with previous recordings to assess the patient's progress. The anaesthetist may have had the patient under deliberate hypotension throughout surgery (to minimise blood loss) and postoperatively careful observation of the blood pressure return to normal is necessary.

Make sure that the patient is warm enough. If the 'halothane shakes' are present increase the oxygen as the patient consumes more oxygen when shivering. The patient's blood pressure may be low because of pain or lack of fluids. Occasionally the blood pressure may be high due to pain; it is difficult trying to decide which but experienced staff are always on hand in the recovery room to help you assess the patient's condition and the need for analgesia.

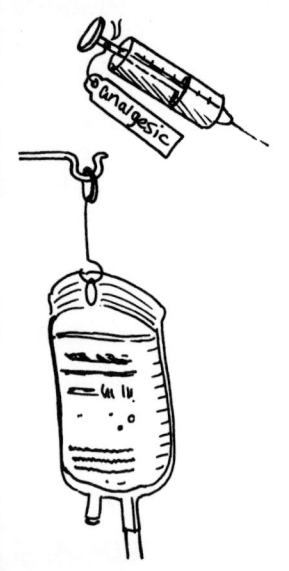

If naloxone has been used at the end of the anaesthetic to reverse any narcotics used then the patient may well be in pain on arrival in the recovery room. Do not be mean with analgesics or feel a statutory length of time should pass before giving any.

The wound dressings and drains are checked for blood loss. If a tourniquet was used during surgery then there may well be a moderate loss immediately postoperation. An assessment of the loss should be noted. Check that the IV is running well and that the catheter is draining. If there is an underwater chest drain ensure that the water level oscillates as the patient breathes.

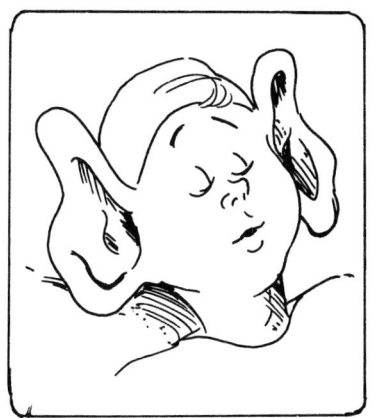

Remember the sense of hearing was the last to go and the first to return so there is no need to shout at patients. The sound is distorted to them and combined with pinching and other nasty waking up devices is an unpleasant way to rouse a patient.

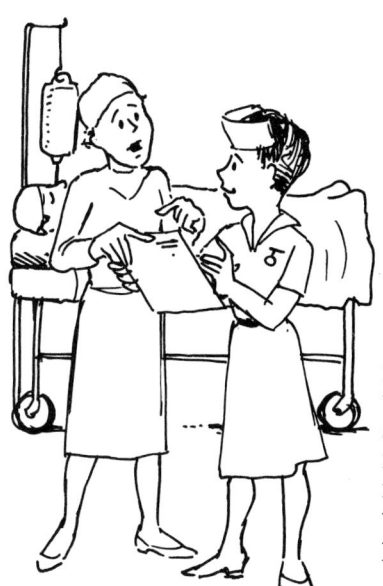

Patients are *never* left alone in the recovery room. There is always a risk of inhalation of vomit. Most patients stay at least an hour postoperatively to ensure that they are comfortable, their vital signs are stable, IV running, that any monitoring needed is within normal limits and that dressings and drains are satisfactory. If there is any doubt at all the anaesthetist must be kept informed and he will see the patient before he/she is returned to the ward. It is important to inform the ward nurse of all relevant details when she comes to collect the patient.

RESPIRATORY OR CARDIAC ARREST
Sound the alarm and a free anaesthetist will come. You have the resuscitation trolley, drugs and equipment all to hand. Suction the patient and use the 'Ambu' (self-reflating) bag until an anaesthetist comes and then follow his directions as in any arrest procedure.

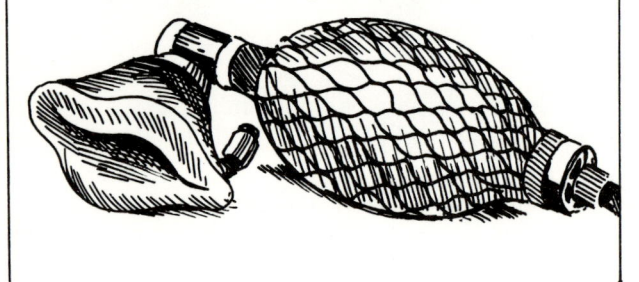

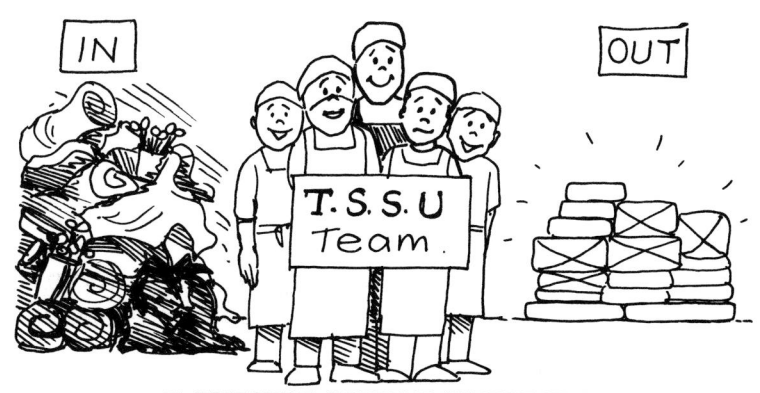

7. THEATRE STERILE SUPPLY UNIT

If you think theatre is backstage work the trusty souls of the TSSU are at the back of that backstage! They never see the patients at all and yet everything those people do in preparing and cleaning up is with patient safety in mind. The TSSU staff are divided into two teams: one team works on collection of used equipment and its cleaning, the other on assembly of trays, wrapping and autoclaving.

When used equipment, rubbish and dirty linen are collected from the disposal area the TSSU staff wear protective gloves and aprons. This minimises the risk of potential infection to themselves. Rubbish is placed ready for incineration and linen for the laundry, but this is not collected for a couple of hours to allow time for a search for missing items. Dirty instruments are opened, washed and cleaned (by hand for delicate telescopes and eye, neuro and cardiovascular instruments) or by machine or ultrasonic cleaners. The instruments are then lubricated and dried.

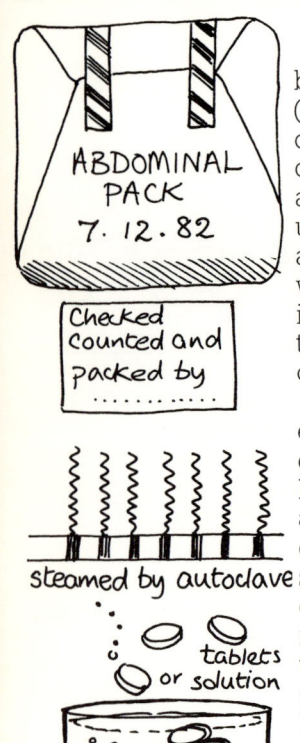

As the set of instruments is assembled it is checked for anything missing (and the theatre staff alerted) and for its correct functioning. The trays are then covered with fresh linen and repacked according to a list so the sets are always uniform. A second count is then made and a ticket placed on the tray stating who made the set and counted it, thus identifying the person responsible to the scrub nurse should she find a discrepancy.

Particular care has to be taken with extremely expensive telescopes, fibre optic equipment and fine instruments. Many of these instruments cannot be autoclaved and must be sterilised by other methods, e.g. glutaraldehyde solutions, formalin tablets and vapour, ethylene oxide, hot air oven, gamma irradiation, etc. While working in TSSU the different methods of sterilisation of equipment will be explained. You will learn how you can achieve sterility of objects by varying the temperature and pressure at which heat is applied; how effective the solution methods are and the various hazards and disadvantages of each system. For example, autoclaving blunts sharp instruments, ruins telescopes and light cords, and melts plastic equipment. Ethylene oxide is poisonous, needs hours of aeration and permeates plastics and silicones to their detriment. Gamma irradiation sterilises implants and delicate equipment perfectly, but it is impracticable in a hospital set-up.

INSTRUMENTS

When learning sets of instruments don't panic and be put off by the different names. *Know anatomy*. If you understand the different layers of tissue the surgeon will find as he dissects, you will be able to hand him the appropriate instruments:

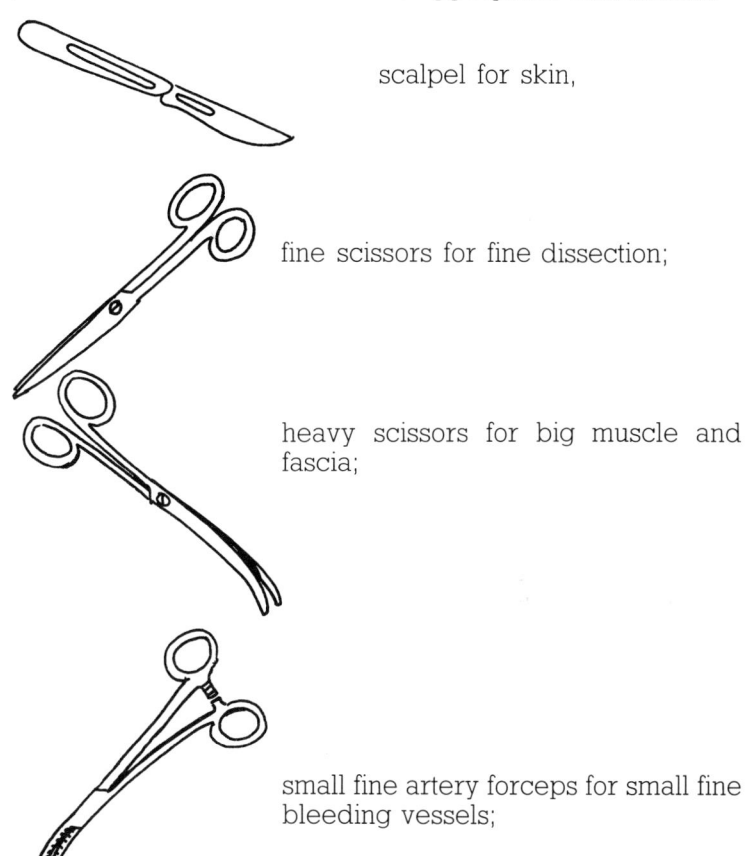

scalpel for skin,

fine scissors for fine dissection;

heavy scissors for big muscle and fascia;

small fine artery forceps for small fine bleeding vessels;

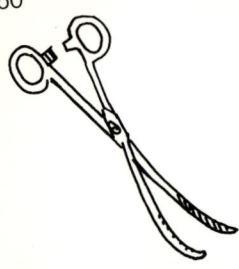

and artery forceps that are long and go round corners for bleeders that are deep and round corners (the gallbladder and in the pelvis).

There is no magic about it! *Know the function* of an instrument.

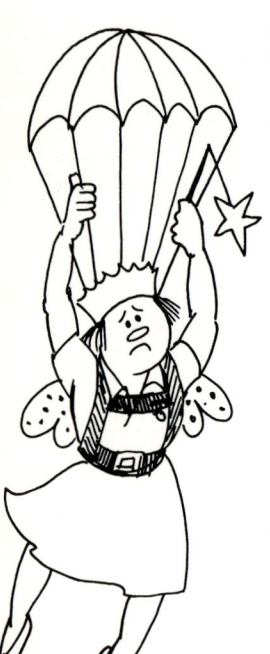

Artery forceps have small serrations for a good grip and a ratchet on the handle to keep that grip.

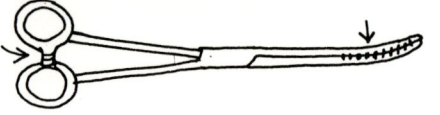

Forceps that have a ratchet but big teeth are obviously not for blood vessels but for tissue holding, e.g. fine and smooth for holding bowel, big and chunky for holding bone.

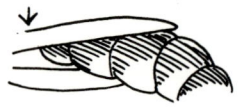

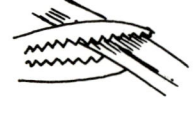

Retractors are of appropriate size for the size of the wound, e.g. fine skin hooks for the face, deep, broad and curved for inside the abdomen. Microscopic instruments are needed for arterial work: inside the brain, the eye and the ear. It's all very logical!

Think through the logical order of the surgery:

Clean up: sponge holders

Towel up: towel clips

Cut: scalpel

Dissect: toothed tissue forceps in one hand, scissors in the other

Haemostasis: artery forceps, diathermy

Visualise the field: retractors

Excise tissue: tissue-holding forceps

Closure: needle holders

There! You've just made your first set of general instruments! Miniaturise this for plastic surgery, babies, etc.; add longer and larger of the same for deep pelvic and thoracic work. Then think of extras for bone surgery: a scraper is needed to scratch periosteum from bone; cutters and nibblers are needed as well as chisels and osteotomes (plus a hammer to make them work) to remove bone. Curved periosteal elevators are for ribs in a thoracotomy set, a fine one in the neuro set for the skull. For surgery in orifices such as the ear, nose and vagina the order is a little changed in that a speculum is needed first, to visualise the field, and then the operating instruments. It doesn't matter who named the equipment, but it is important to learn what it does.

For procedures such as bronchoscopy, cystoscopy or laparoscopy there is still a logical way to think it through.

Clean up
Towel up
Insert tube to hold the:
   Telescope
   Light source
   Water tubing

No need to clean up for a bronchoscopy but the oxygen line not the water line is needed to inflate the patient. In laparoscopy the patient's abdomen is filled with CO_2 (carbon dioxide) before the cannula holding the telescope is passed, but these are variations on the basic theme.

TSSU is also responsible for ordering and storing all the implants. The subject of implants such as heart valves, arterial grafts, artificial hip prostheses and knees, and intra-ocular lenses, is much too vast to start here. You can enjoy asking more about this while working in the unit. More commonly you will be dealing with sutures, as described below.

SUTURES

There are two basic types of suture: absorbable and non-absorbable. Of the absorbable sutures there is catgut (which is actually sheep's gut!) and an artificial polyglycolic suture commonly called by its trade name 'Dexon' (Davis and Geck).

Plain catgut (in yellow packets) lasts about a week and is just for 'tacking' tissue together to allow natural healing to take place (for example, fat). Chromic catgut (in brown packets) has been treated with chromic acid to prolong the absorbing time to about three weeks. This is used to suture together stronger tissue such as muscle. As Dexon is man-made it is of more consistent quality than catgut, does not need storing in a preservative solution and is braided for easier tying. It takes about a month to dissolve and, therefore, is better and safer for patients (for example, the elderly) who will take longer to heal.

Of the non-absorbable sutures there are many types including silk, linen, steel, polyester and nylon. Silk (blue packets) is commonly used but as it is spun by a silkworm it carries an infection risk, rots easily and breaks. Polyester (orange packets) is braided for easy tying and is uniformly stronger than silk (but it is more expensive). Nylon (green packets) causes no tissue reaction and has become popular for skin suturing, but like fishing line it is difficult to tie knots with!

Size 1 and 2 is a very thick suture for chest closure and muscle; through 2/0, 3/0 for internal suturing of bowel or skin; through 5/0, 6/0 for babies and arteries to 10/0 for inside the eye.

Commonly the needles are mounted on to the suture. This 'atraumatic' fusion means only one hole is made and is filled by the suture material. Originally made for bowel surgery so no *E.coli* would spill into the abdomen, the idea is so popular that now virtually all sutures come with needles.

There are two types of needles: cutting and round-bodied.

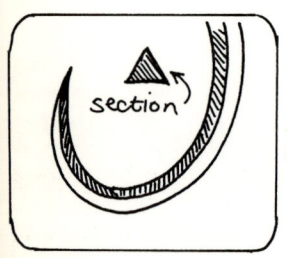

A cutting needle has three sharp edges and is therefore ideal for use on skin.

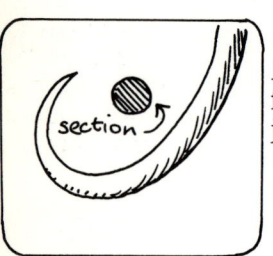

A round-bodied needle is blunt except for its very tip which needs to be sharp just to perforate the tissue.

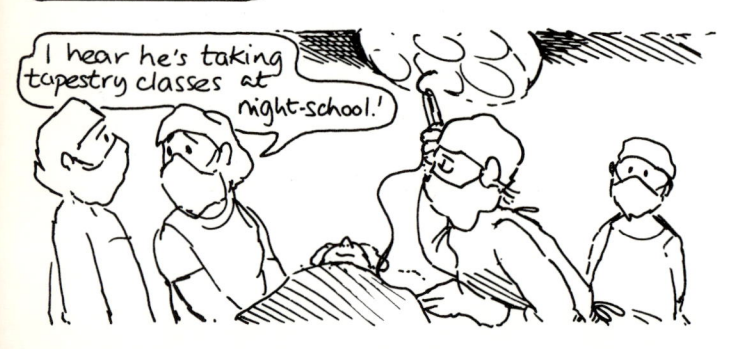

8. CONCLUSION

You have now witnessed a 'thumb-nail sketch' of the theatre team at work. Each one doing their own task for better patient care and safety. You will have the opportunity of witnessing doctors working for prolonged periods and often under stress. At other times you will hear them discuss their ideas on politics or whatever. Hence theatres can be hotbeds of personality clashes! Consider this when you are next in an annoying situation. Concern yourself only with good technique for the patient's safety, keep the surgeon and anaesthetist happy so they work well for the patient, and constantly remember you are the patient's representative to anticipate and care for his/her needs.

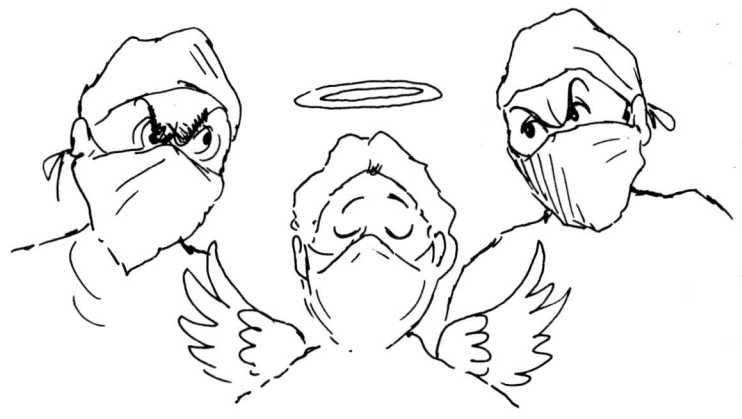

GLOSSARY

Anastomosis:	join together
Angio:	arterial
Arthro:	joint
Cardio	heart
Chole:	gallbladder
Cranio:	skull
Cysto:	bladder
Derma:	skin
Desis:	fuse, fix
Docho	duodenum
Ectomy:	remove
Endo:	inside
Gastro	stomach
Gram:	picture
Hyst:	uterus
Mast:	breast
Nephro:	kidney
Neuro:	nerve
Ooph:	ovary
Opth	eye
Oro:	mouth
Orrhaphy:	repair
Ortho:	bone
Oscopy:	to look
Otomy:	to cut a hole
Plasty:	renew
Pneumo:	lung
Resection:	remove part

APPENDIX: OUTLINE OF THE RECOMMENDED SYLLABUS

The syllabus extends for about eight weeks.

AIMS

The syllabus aims to enable the student nurse to:
(1) participate with understanding in the total care of the surgical patient;
(2) care for the patient in the preoperative, intraoperative and postoperative period.

OBJECTIVES

The objectives are to teach skills to the student nurse in the areas described below.

Care of the patient in the anaesthetic room
Preparation of the basic equipment and drugs. The procedure for the reception, identification and special needs of the patient. Establishing an immediate rapport with the patient in order to allay anxiety. Create a quiet environment. Respect the dignity of the patient and be aware of the danger of careless remarks. Care for the conscious and unconscious patient and hazards to the anaesthetised patient.

Care of the patient in the operating theatre
Preparation, use and care of basic equipment. Participate as a member of the surgical team, fulfilling the duties of the anaesthetic, circulating or scrub nurse. Utilise correctly theatre apparel. Prepare, store, dispense and dispose of sterile items. Scrub up. Gown and gloves. Handle instruments. Handle ligatures and sutures. Prepare sterile equipment. Correctly drape the instrument trolley and the patient. Maintain the sterile field. Knowledge of anatomy and physiology. Hazards of equipment and atmospheric pollution. Principles of aseptic technique and

sources of infection. The correct procedure for lifting, transferring and positioning the patient. The operating table and the attachments. Receive, label and correctly despatch specimens. Apply the correct lines of internal, external, emergency and interpersonal communications. Methods of recording information and its legal implications. Appreciate the team work necessary for successful patient care. Be aware of the stresses which may arise and their effect on staff and patient care.

Care of the patient in the recovery room
Maintain the patient's airway. Observe and record data. Report changes in the patient's clinical condition. Know the stages of recovery. Know the resuscitation techniques and equipment. Administer oxygen, drugs and IV therapy as prescribed. Use of suction apparatus. The importance of communication between theatre and ward staff for continued patient care.

The Recommended Syllabus for Student and Pupil Nurse Training in the Operating Theatre 1977 is published by The National Association of Theatre Nurses, 22 Mount Parade, Harrogate, HG1 1BV.

USEFUL ADDRESSES

AUSTRALIA: Australian Confederation of Operating Room Nurses, P.O. Box 326, Freemantle 6160, West Australia

BOLIVIA: The President, Asociación Nacional de Enfermeras Profesionales de Bolivia, Srta. Rogelia Salinas Aracena, Hospital de Clínicas, Casilla 249, La Paz

BRAZIL: Associaçao Brasileira de Enfermagem, Av. L-2 Norte, Módulo B. Quadra 603, CEP 70.830, Brasilia

BURMA (Union of): Burma Nurses Association, c/o The Lady Health Visitors' Training School, 11 East Bazaar Road, Rangoon

CANADA: Canadian Nurses Association, 50 The Driveway, Ottawa, K2P 1E2, Ontario

CZECHOSLOVAKIA: Czech Nurses Society, Jihozapadni V. 1023, 141 00, Praha 4, Sporilov, CSSR

DENMARK: The Danish Nurses' Organization, P.O. Box 1084, DK-1008, Copenhagen K

EGYPT: Egyptian Nurses Syndicate, 5 Sarai Street, Manial, Cairo

FRANCE: Association Nationale Française des Infirmières et Infirmiers Diplômés et Eléves (ANFIIDE), Avenue de la République 24, F-75011, Paris

GERMANY (Federal Republic): Deutscher Berufsverband für Krankenpflege, Arndstrasse 15, D-6000, Frankfurt/Main 1

GHANA: Ghana Registered Nurses Association, P.O. Box 2994, Accra

GUYANA: Guyana Nurses Association, 178 Alexander and Charlotte Streets, Lacytown, Georgetown

HONG KONG: The Hong Kong Nurses Association, 12th Floor, Hyde Centre, Flats A-D, 221-226 Gloucester Road, Wanchai, Hong Kong

HUNGARY: Nursing Committee of the Hungarian Hospital Federation, Postafíók 54, 1027 Budapest 114

INDIA: Trained Nurses Association of India, L-17 Green Park, New Delhi 110016

ISRAEL: The National Association of Nurses in Israel, The Histadrut, 93 Arlosoroff Street, Tel Aviv

ITALY: Consociazione Nazionale delle Associazioni Infermiere-Infermieri ad altri Operatori Sanitario-Sociali, Via Arno 62, I-00198, Roma

JAPAN: Japanese Nursing Association, 8-2, 5-chome, Jinguamae, Shibuya-ku, Tokyo

KENYA: National Nurses Association of Kenya, P.O. Box 49422, Nairobi

KOREA (South): Korean Nurses Association, 88-7 Sang Lim Dong, Choong Ku, Seoul

MALAYSIA: Malaysian Nurses Association, School of Nursing, General Hospital, Kuala Lumpur

NETHERLANDS: National Nurses Association, Frans Halsstraat 23, 2021 EG Haarlem

NEW ZEALAND: New Zealand Nurses' Association, Inc., C.P.O. Box 2128, Wellington

NIGERIA: The National Association of Nigeria Nurses and Midwives, P.O. Box 3857, Ikeja Post Office, Lagos

NORWAY: Norwegian Nurses Association, Postboks 3649, Gamlebyen-Oslo 1

PAKISTAN: Pakistan Nurses Federation, C/O College of Nursing, Jinnah Postgraduate Medical Centre, Karachi

PHILIPPINES: Philippine Nurses Association, 1663 Kansas Avenue, Malate, Manila, D-2801

SPAIN: Consejo General de Ayudantes Técnicos Sanitarios y Diplomados en Enfermería, Buen Suceso 6-20, Madrid 8

SRI LANKA: Sri Lanka Nurses Association, Room 123, Nurses Home, 93 Regent Street, Colombo 10

SUDAN: Sudan Professional Nurses Association, P.O. Box 1472, Khartoum

SWEDEN: Swedish Nurses Association, P.O. Box 5277, S-102 46, Stockholm 5

SWITZERLAND: Association Suisse des Infirmières et Infirmiers, Secrétariat Central, Choisystrasse 1, CH-3008, Bern; and International Council of Nurses, P.O. Box 42, 1211 Geneva 20

TANZANIA: Tanzania Registered Nurses' Association, P.O. Box 4357, Dar-es-Salaam

THAILAND: The Nurses Association of Thailand, 21/12 Soi Rang Nam, Rajchaprarob Road, Bangkok

TURKEY: Turkish Nurses Association, Türk Hemsireler Dernegi Genel Merkezi, Saglik Sokak No. 36/4, Ankara

UNITED KINGDOM: The Royal College of Nursing of the United Kingdom, 1 Henrietta Place, Cavendish Square, London, W1M 0AB

UNITED STATES OF AMERICA: American Operating Room Nurses, 10170 East Mississippi Avenue, Denver, Colorado 80231

YUGOSLAVIA: Nurses Association of Yugoslavia, Mlinarska 34, 41000 Zagreb

INDEX

Airway, 10, 18, 53
Alarms
  cardiac arrest, 52
  equipment, 9, 14, 27
  patient, 14
Ambu bag, 56
Anaesthetic drugs, 10, 20
Anaesthetic machine, 9
Anaesthetic mask, 10
Anaesthetic nurse, 7, 16, 18, 46
Anaesthetic room, 8, 9, 16, 17
Analgesia, 21, 54
Arterial line, 13

Cardiac arrest, 25, 50, 56
Catgut, *see* Sutures
Circulating nurse, 26, 27, 37, 46-51
Colour codes
  equipment, 9
  uniform, 4
Counting, 37, 43
Cricoid pressure, 18, 19
CVP (central venous pressure) recording, 13

Defibrillator, 25
Diathermy, 15, 27, 40, 46, 47
Disposal
  instruments, 45, 51, 57
  laundry, 45, 51, 57
  rubbish, 9, 45, 51, 57
  sharps, 44, 45

Draping, 36, 45

Elephant tubing, 9, 10
Endotracheal tube, 11-13, 15, 18, 19, 22, 51
Epidural, 23

Gloving, 33-35
Gowning, 32, 33

'Halothane shakes', 54
Hepatitis, 9, 47

Induction, 18-21
Infection, 3, 7, 10, 43, 45, 47, 51, 57
Instrument count, 37, 43
Instrument sets, 58-62
Instruments
  care of, 57, 58
  cleaning of, 57, 58
  setting up, 40
Intubation, 11-13, 18, 19, 22

Laryngoscope, 11, 18
Local anaesthetic, 24

Medical treatment, 49
Monitors
  equipment, 14
  patient, 13, 19

Narcotics, 20, 21
Needles, *see* Sutures

Pin index, 9
Policies, 6
Pollution, 14
Positioning pads, 14
Premedication, 17, 20

Rebreathing bag, 10
Reception, 7
Recovery observations, 53-55
Recovery room, 52
Regional anaesthesia, 23
Register of operations, 45
Relaxants, 18, 20, 22
Respiratory arrest, 56
Reversants, 20, 23, 51, 54
'Runner', *see* Circulating nurse

Scalpel blades
　disposal, 44
　mounting, 38
Scrubbing procedure, 29-31
Scrub nurse, 28, 36-45
Specimens, 44, 48
Sterilisation methods, 58
Stress, 65
Suction, 9, 18, 27, 47, 51, 53
Sutures, 38, 42, 43, 62-64

Swabs
   counting, 37, 43
   disposal, 47
   mounting, 41
Syllabus, 67, 68

Throat pack, 12
TSSU (Theatre Sterile Supply Unit), 57, 58

Vaporiser, 9
Ventilation
   of patient, 11
   of theatre, 26